Maggie Tisserand & Monika Jünemann

The Magic and Power
of Lavender

The Secret of Its Fragrance
and Practical Application
in Health Care and Cosmetics

D0035696

LOTUS LIGHT
SHANGRI-LA

Although this book offers a variety of tools for treating minor ailments, it is not meant to give recommendations or advice for the treatment of specific illnesses. When ill, it is suggested that you consult a physician or qualified holistic health practitioner.

The authors

2nd printing 1996

1. American Edition 1994
© by Lotus Light Publications
PO Box 325
Twin Lakes, WI 53181
The Shangri-La series is published
in cooperation with Schneelöwe Verlagsberatung,
Federal Republic of Germany
English Translation: Matthias Dehne
Originally published 1989
by Windpferd Verlagsgesellschaft
© by Schneelöwe Verlagsberatung,
8955 Aitrang, Federal Republic of Germany

ISBN 0-941524-88-4

Printed in the USA

2

Contents

Acknowledgements

Grateful thanks go to all those people who have responded with such positive enthusiasm to requests for information.

Henry Head, Norfolk Lavender
Mr Denny, Bridestowe Estate
Robert Carberry, Quintessence Perfumes Ltd
Hazel Ransome, William Ransome Ltd
David Christie, The Jersey Lavender Farm
Pat Moody, Brighton Polytechnic Library

and special thanks to Sue Robinson and Melanie Barrass for their editing skills on the English edition.

Maggie Tisserand

Acknowledgements

Many people throughout history have devoted their lives to the service of health and to the cultivation and application of lavender. Without their efforts this book could not have been written. I wish to thank them all.

I am very grateful to Maggie Tisserand for the inspiration and ideas she shared with me during the all too few days in which we first discussed co-authoring this book, and for the energy she gave - an energy which manifests in single-minded pursuit of a worthy goal.

I would like to thank Matthias Dehne for the research he undertook for us in the *New York Public Library* and the *Bavarian State Library* in Munich and for translating my part of the manuscript into English and Maggie's part into German. Grateful thanks also go to Asta Skocir for her special contribution.

I am greatly obliged to my husband, Wolfgang Junemann, for his untiring and always positively challenging support that gave me the strength to complete my work, and I have to thank my daughter Jennifer for her understanding and for giving me the breathing space I needed.

Many thanks also go to Mr Linder and Mr Schierholz.

Monika Jünemann

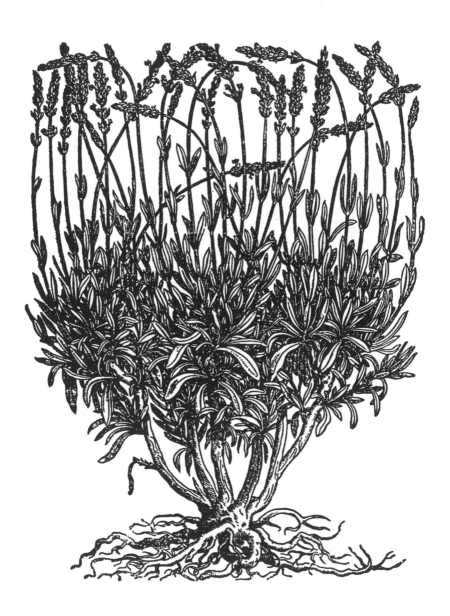

Preface

Aromatherapy is such an integral part of my life that for me to quantify its value would be to attempt the near impossible. I have so many reasons to be grateful for the therapeutic properties of essential oils, especially in their contribution to the health of my three children. The essence to which I particularly owe a great debt is lavender, and it is for this reason that I am delighted to be co-author of this book.

I first encountered lavender in 1972 when I was living in a "medical commune" in South London with a group of people studying various aspects of "alternative" medicine. Amongst them was Robert Tisserand who was researching aromatherapy and others who were learning massage, reflexology, homeopathy and radiesthesia.

One day a friend appeared at the door with a badly burned arm. Beefy, his nickname, had taken the cap from his radiator and the boiling steam had removed the skin from his wrist to his elbow. He was in excruciating pain but refused to go to hospital and asked us to look after him. I gave him a dose of homeopathic arnica to combat the shock. With sterile instruments, Annie, who was a state registered nurse, carefully removed the dead skin from what she regarded as a second degree burn. Robert then sprinkled neat lavender oil onto sterile gauze and applied it to the burn. The lavender stung for a few minutes but then quickly cooled the burned skin and lessened the pain. Lavender was used in this way every day for just over a week, and at no time did the burn become infected. Within two weeks the arm had healed completely, leaving no scar whatsoever, and Beefy returned to work.

Until this time I had been studying homeopathy, for which I had enormous respect, when suddenly I was shown that the healing power of essential oils was also truly wonderful -almost, one might say, miraculous. I did not know then that Robert's choice of lavender was based on his knowledge that Gattefossé had, in 1930, burned his hand in a laboratory explosion and healed it with lavender oil, or that Dr Valnet had used lavender to treat burns with equally remarkable results. I only knew that I had just been an eye witness to an incredible incident; one which left me with a profound feeling of awe and respect for lavender, and for aromatherapy as a whole.

Over the years I have used lavender in many different ways for treating a variety of problems and conditions, and although lavender is just one of a large number of essences in regular use, it remains, for me the most versatile and reliable of essences. Lavender is gentle on the skin and soothing to the emotions and yet possesses a power in its action at least equal to that of antibiotics and tranquillizing drugs.

If I add to my praise of lavender my appreciation of its beautiful and enchanting aroma, then I have to say, in short, that lavender makes a very important contribution to the health and well-being of humanity.

From the bottom of my heart I give thanks to the Creator for this wonderful gift.

Maggie Tisserand

Foreword

Our common interest in aromatherapy brought us together. Since the "personal chemistry" seemed to be just right, Maggie and I decided quite spontaneously to co-author this book on the magic and power of lavender, one of the most adaptable essences with its familiar and well-loved fragrance.

Our main goal is to introduce you to the delightful and enticing secrets of this plant and its essence. We wish to demonstrate its healing power, familiarise you with its long and fascinating history and present to you the places and people involved in its cultivation. We sincerely hope that our efforts will make you well acquainted with this lovely plant, and, should you already be familiar with it, make you appreciate it even more for its many most wonderful qualities.

We have asked doctors, holistic health practitioners, chemists, perfumers, and friends bout their experiences with the "blue flower", and we take this opportunity to share our own observations with you.

May the wings of lavender's charming fragrance uplift you, and may our practical suggestions enrich your lives. We hope from now on, you will be in a position to truly enjoy lavender and its essence.

Monika Jünemann

Introduction

The lavender plant has been known for centuries, and since time immemorial man has used lavender to relax, soothe and refresh. The scent of lavender, in a way, has permeated whole regions of Europe, contributing to their special character, and it has dominated perfumery for most of its history. To this very day lavender has remained one of the most familiar, popular and utilised of all fragrances.

Ancient medical texts extol its healing powers. From the history of the Middle Ages, we learn that people handling lavender never fell victim to the bubonic plague. Moreover, when inhaled regularly, lavender could also protect against tuberculosis.

Other uses have been known. In ancient Egypt the priests are said to have dipped linen sheets in lavender essence and natural asphalt in preparation for mummifying corpses. Without the essential oil of lavender Joseph Niepce would not have succeeded in taking the first photograph, his so-called heliogram, obtained after he had coated a silver plate with bitumen (a natural asphalt) diluted with lavender oil. And of course, many poets and writers have praised the wonders of lavender in their writing.

Today medical science and chemistry have found conclusive evidence that the healing powers of this sweet-smelling essence have been praised for good reasons. Far from being unfounded superstitions, the old myths and traditions represent valid knowledge and experience.

Lavender enchants us, beckoning us to open up to its seductive messages. It offers its powers for us to recognise and use in the promotion of health, beauty and well-being. It has the power to create harmony where harmony is required. It does so without violence or force. On the contrary, its ways are rather gentle and subtle. It may touch our bodies and souls either through our skin or, with the air that we breathe, through our sense of smell. Meandering through complex pathways, it reaches its final destination - the nerve centre where our emotional memories are stored. Though they can rightfully be called ethereal, lavender's effects are nevertheless recognizable, and modern medical science has succeeded in analysing them.

In connection with the growing popularity of essential oils, the knowledge of their use, and their therapeutic properties, one name has to be mentioned above all: René-Maurice Gattefossé who, in 1928, founded modern aromatherapy. Even the word "aromatherapy" is his creation. In Gattefossé's life, lavender played a crucial role in that it guided him to venture in a new direction. One day, Gattefossé scalded his hand whilst working in his laboratory and instinctively immersed it in pure lavender oil. The burn healed much quicker than expected, leaving no scars at all, and this remarkable event inspired him to devote all his energies for the rest of his life to the scientific exploration of essential oils and their properties. Many others followed in his footsteps to broaden and substantiate his initial findings, making available to us an ancient art of healing in modern form.

However, aromatherapy takes us beyond our usual understanding of the word "therapy", namely the treating of diseases or disorders by medical or physical means. Aromatherapy is preventive care, and in this sense opens up a whole new way of life to us. By strengthening our immune system, it can thwart attacks on our physical and mental well-being. Since, through the use of essential oils, we are strengthened, disease cannot take root. Aromatherapy moves through all our senses to benefit body and mind, affecting all facets of our existence: the organs and their functions, our emotions, our thinking, even our looks.

We sincerely believe in the effectiveness of such an holistic approach, and the aim of this book is to make a contribution to the overall well-being of our readers.

We wish to introduce to them the miraculously versatile lavender plant and its essential oil. Lavender can be used in so many ways. Lavender oil can be added to baths, lotions, massage oils, perfumes, potpourries, sachets, aroma lamps (essential oil burners) and so forth. But we also shall make some suggestions as to how doctors or non-medical practitioners may find this essence useful.

The active substances of lavender oil can enhance the quality of our lives, and their enchanting scent fill us with joy. Nobody likes foul smells. Only sweet fragrances can give wings to our imagination.

The Use of Lavender in Ancient Times

We don't know exactly where lvender originated. Different sources point in different directions: Persia, Egypt, Greece, Italy. Whoever first enjoyed lavender and its many healing properties, cannot be determined with absolute certainty.

To our knowledge, its history begins some time during the first century A.D. when the Roman physician of Greek descent, Pedanios Dioscurides, mentioned "Oil of Spike or Stoechaeus"* in his "Materia Medica" a "seminal achievement" in the true sense of the word. Even in seventeenth century Europe this "Materia Medica" was still in use in an updated and extensively revised edition.

It is probable that Dioscurides' "spike and stoechaeus" oils were not essential oils but infused oils. Infused oils are made by placing a quantity of the dried plant material into a vessel, and completely covering the herb with a fatty oil such as olive or almond. The vessel is made water-tight and placed in a pan of hot water and simmered for an hour or two. When cool, th Wromatic oil" is filtered to remove particles of plant and stored in an airtight container. Infused o of lavender would have been used

---

*The botanical names in use today are *Lavendula Spica* and *Lavendula angustifolia-stoechas*. The designation '*Lavendula*' is derived from the Italian and common usage since the late Middle Ages.

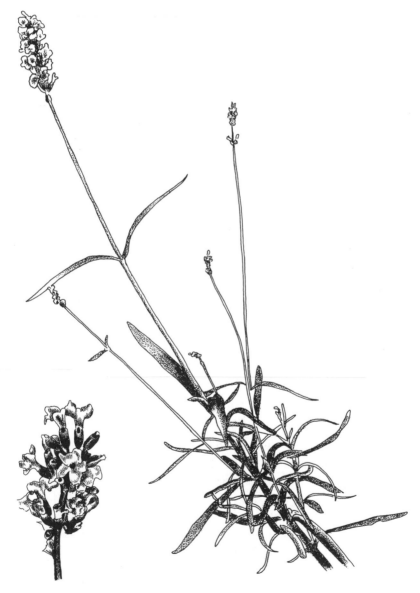

for massage of painful joints, muscular aches and to promote healing during illness.

The fine art of distillation was first described in 550 A.D. by the Byzantine physician Aetius of Amida, and approximately five hundred years later by the Arab philosopher and physician Ibn Sina, better known in the West as Avicenna. Avicenna's "Canon Medicinae" gives a number of prescriptions involving the use of essential oils. Like Dioscurides' "Materia Medica" the "Canon Medicinae" in its Latin translation influenced European medicine for many centuries and was widely taught at universities throughout the continent. It was the most comprehensive treatise on medicine of its time, serving as a textbook of physiology, pathology, diagnosis and treatment, and including psychological advice, diet, exercise, herbal prescriptions, essential oils and even surgery.

Regarding the distribution of *Lavendula stoechas*, several facts lead us to assume that the plant might have been brought to the south of France around 500 B.C., when Greek colonists first settled in the area of Marseilles. Situated between St Tropez and Toulon, the resort town of Le Lavendou still exists today opposite the small islands known as Iles d'Hyères. In ancient times these islands were called "Stoechades" and were completely covered with lavender plants.

During the Middle Ages the knowledge and lore of the healing arts were preserved by monks, particularly those of the Benedictine order. In Germany the name "lavindula" first appears in a prescription dating from the ninth century, though the older name of "spike" was used more frequently. In the course of the twelfth century the abbess Hildegard von Bingen (1100-1179) devoted an entire chapter ("de lavandulare") in one of her works to the plant. Apart from Hildegard in Germany, no other medieval author seems to have said much about its use. Albert Magnus, drawing on Avicenna, mentions its fragrance just once, Ortlof praises its healing effects on "ailments of the womb", and Hyronimus Bock derives the name from Latin "lavare" (to wash), because lavender, then as now, was added to the baths. In the famous collection of herbal remedies "Gart der Gesundheit" ("Garden of Health") which appeared in 1485, lavender is called the "plant of the Virgin Mary" and much praised for its supposed ability to dispel the "desires of the flesh".

In the 1500s lavender gained much wider appeal, mainly because the art of distillation was rediscovered from Graeco-Roman sources. In his "Dispensatorium Noricum" which appeared in Paris in 1543, Valerius Cordus speaks of three oils: turpentine, juniper and spike. In a revised edition of the same work, which appeared forty years later, *oleum lavendulae* is mentioned as well. A study on distillation was soon to follow. Compiled by Gaultherus Ryff the "New and Extensive Book of Distillation" describes in detail how in Southern France lavender oil was obtained from lavender plants, with the observation that "it fetches very high a price indeed".

More significant than any of the aforementioned books was a book by Paracelsus called "Elixirs and Fragrances". Nostrodamus, an orthodox doctor practising unorthodox medicine, was influenced by this book which probably gave him the courage to work with the victims of the plague, "le charbon". While ministering to plague victims from Marseilles to Lyons, his only protection was to eat "rose pills" and to carry a dispenser containing fragrant materials and oils, one of which was lavender. Distillation grew even more fashionable as the sixteenth passed into the seventeenth century. In Haute Provence, wild lavender was cut regularly. But lavender was also grown and harvested near Vienna and later, on a much grander scale, in Surrey (Mitcham) and Norfolk in England.

The tolerance for "bad smells" which had prevailed during the late Middle Ages was on the wane. Fragrance was the word of the day, and fragrant substances in all forms had their renaissance. Henry VIII and his daughter Elizabeth I contributed to this development, and so did Sir Walter Raleigh and Sir Francis Bacon. Everyone knows about their impact on the shaping of modern Europe, but few know that they also enriched the history of scent. Through their example they popularized the use of fragrances and oils. In Paris the first perfumery store opened to the public, and in better class English households people distilled their own fragrant substances.

A recent visit to the famous lavender fields in Norfolk revealed that lavender has been cultivated there since the mid-sixteenth century. Henry VIII had beds of lavender planted around the garden of the castle where Elizabeth I played as a child. She came to love herb gardens, and lavender in particular. During her own reign herb gardens gained a popularity they had never enjoyed before and shall probably never attain again. In larger mansions and estates, special servants were assigned to the "stillroom" to take care of the lotions and pomanders for their masters and mistresses.

For more than two centuries lively English lavender, cheerful and fresh, remained the favourite scent. The fairer sex, fastidious women of all ages, literally bathed in lavender water to protect themselves against "foul smells" and the "swoons". Lavender was dried and used in sachets. Put under the pillow, these sachets were supposed to fight off migraine and to promote rejuvenating sleep. Sir Hugh Plat describes the many uses of lavender water in his book "Delights for Ladies" of 1609, but he also warns against its "hot and subtle spirit".

The French were less puritanical than the English. In France women were adored for their beauty. Nothing serves to illustrate this better than the story of Ninon de Lenclos (also known as Anne de Lanclos). Born in 1520 she lived an exciting, some might say scandalous, life as an accomplished courtesan and was also the lover and confidante of the playwright, Molière. Even in her later years she succeeded in keeping her body slim and her skin fresh and free of wrinkles and died a well-preserved 85 years of age! She revealed only a few of her countless beauty secrets, one of which was a herb bath: "Sprinkle one handful of each dried lavender, rosemary, mint, crushed comfrey root, and thyme in a bowl, pour half a pint of boiling water over the herbs, and let them steep for twenty minutes. Add the mixture to the bathwater and sit in the tub for twenty minutes."

As a more hygienic lifestyle definitely became the trend of the times, lavender oil quickly occupied pride of place amongst essential oils. One event may have played a crucial role in this development. We are referring to the "remedy" that, as early as 1508, was concocted in the newly established laboratory of Santa Maria Novella, just outside the city walls of Florence, Italy. Secretly passed on from one generation to the next, this prescription became famous after 1710 under its new name "Eau de Cologne 4711". In those days it was used not only as a beauty or hygiene product but as a "remedy" as well.

Thus we can see that lavender has been used in pharmacy and perfumery almost since time immemorial. Its effectiveness has been proved, and its popularity always maintained.

How Lavender and Perfume Together Made History

Over the centuries the scent of lavender never lost its appeal. However, like all of history, its history is marked by changes of fortune.Favourite fragrances tend to be a reflection of the prevailing spirit of an era. Consequently lavender, though always in use, could not always remain fashionable.

Its career in perfumery started in Paris in the house of René le Florentin, perfumer to Catherine de Medici, the wife of King Henry II of France. As his name suggests, René had indeed come from Florence. In 1533 he opened a perfumery, which quickly gained great popularity, on Rue du Pont-au-Change. Because René's creations unfailingly appealed to the taste of his contemporaries this venture was successful in all respects.

However, times changed; the Age of Enlightenment came, and with it a certain prejudice against sensual perception and sensual delight. The sweet smell of lavender was censored by reason and banished by a mind that valued only those things it considered functional and practical. Nevertheless, once kindled, the desire for sweet smells could not be suppressed completely.

Thus, in 1775 Houbigant was able to open his famous perfumery shop "La Corbeille des Fleurs" situated on Rue St Honoré. Here, among pomades, sachets, essences and perfumes, a mixture of lavender and turpentine oils was sold (pure lavender oil was not yet available). Fragrances experienced another boom, and the more puritan mood of the French Revolution of 1789 hindered, but did not halt, their progress. During the ensuing Napoleonic era perfumes were appreciated as never before, and even animal based fragrances gained acceptance.

Empress Josephine, for example, always wore musk perfume. When Bonaparte left her because she couldn't provide the heir to the throne he so much desired, she strove at least to remain unforgettable. She had the walls of her palace in Malmaison impregnated with musk, a powerful aphrodisiac. Poor Napoleon! In order to escape its effects he literally had to pour Cologne over himself. He even drank it. The pacifying effect of the lavender oil contained in the Cologne secured his releases from Josephine's clutches, which, because of his genuine love for her, was difficult enough without the musk.

In Germany heavy fragrances based on animal related substances were disdained. Here, scents were supposed to suggest freshness and cleanliness. Natural herbaceous fragrances, above all lavender imported from France, were preferred, particularly after the Biedermeier era began in 1815.

The first famous perfume in the history of scent is the so-called "Hungary Water" which originated in 1370 as a distillate of rosemary and was later completed with lavender and marjoram essences. Almost four centuries passed before the next famous name in perfumery was established, again with lavender oil as one of its main ingredients: "Eau de Cologne". Originally used for its antiseptic effects, it contained a mixture of citrus and herbaceous oils and later became the most popular eau de toilette throughout the world.

Eau de Cologne

lavender	1 fl oz
bergamot	1 fl oz
lemon	1 fl oz
orange flower	1 fl oz
cinnamon	1/4 fl oz
rosemary	1/4 fl oz
alcohol (70%)	2 1/2 gallons

The position of Eau de Cologne remained unchallenged for 170 years until the end of the nineteenth century when the "Golden Age" of perfumery dawned, and perfumery became a highly sophisticated art. In the ancient civilisations of Egypt and Mesopotamia and throughout Graeco-Roman history only natural fragrances were known. This continued to be the case until the late nineteenth century. However, with the emergence of organic chemistry, synthetic fragrances were added to the already wide range of existing scents. Now the possibilities were limitless. The year 1882 marked the birth of "Fougère Royale" by Houbigant - another famous perfume with lavender oil as one of its main ingredients.

Thus the essential oil of lavender has indeed been an essential and pervasive element in the history of scent - from time immemorial to this very day.

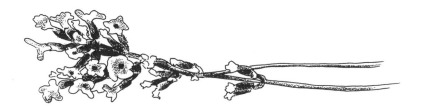

How the Essential Oil Is Obtained from Lavender Plants

"Without distillation no essential oil" - this concise statement sums up how crucial the process of distillation really is. Of course, there are methods other than distillation to obtain aromatic substances, among them extraction, which was used in ancient times before the process of distillation had been discovered. The possible forms of application for extracts, however, are strictly limited. Infused oils are ideal for massage. However, extracts cannot fulfil the many and varied functions of distilled essences: they cannot be used internally, they cannot be used in baths and perfumes and so on.

History of Distillation

Over the centuries the techniques of distillation have been refined in order to secure the maximum yield of essential oil. It has taken a long time to reach this point, and we are indebted to the many generations of researchers and practitioners who have

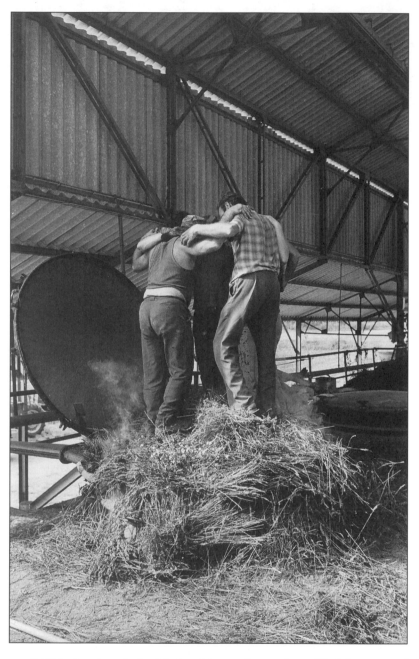

Still being loaded with freshly cut lavender which is pressed in tightly

made the essences available to us. Without their efforts we would not be able to enjoy essential oils as we do, and aromatherapy would be no more than a vague possibility.

We have to reach back into history to find the beginnings of the art of distillation. Primitive devices for distillation were in use as early as 1500-1000 B.C. in both India and China.

In Egypt the tradition is even older, dating back approximately to 4000 B.C. This ancient knowledge was transmitted via Greece and the Roman Empire to the Arabian world where it was developed further during the heyday of Arabian culture in the tenth and eleventh centuries. Later it spread to countries further north.

In the course of the fifteenth century, when pharmacology and the art of healing started to follow separate paths, distillation became established in Europe. Hyronimus Breunschwig of Strassbourg described distillation in 1512 in these apt words which sum up beautifully the actual process and its underlying philosophical principles:

To distill means to separate the subtle
from the coarse, and the coarse from the subtle,
to render the fragile and breakable unbreakable,
to transform the material into the immaterial
the physical into the spiritual
and to beautify what is in need of beautification.

More and more different oils were distilled, but it was not until the nineteenth century that distillation finally produced all the oils that we know today.

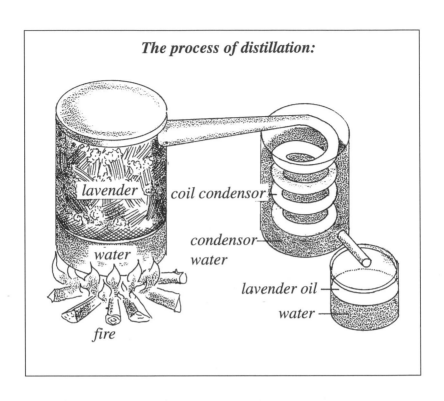

The process of distillation:

lavender

coil condensor

water

condensor water

lavender oil

water

fire

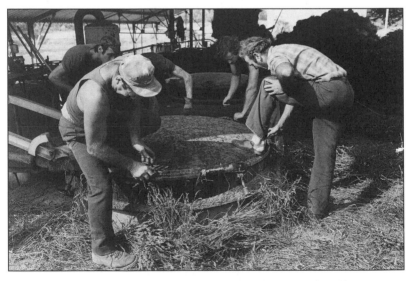

After the lid has been placed on the still, steam distillation may begin

Different Methods to Separate the Subtle from the Coarse

The essential oil of lavender is contained in the flowers, leaves and stems of the plant. Therefore the whole lavender plant is distilled. However, there are also pure flower distillates of lavender used in perfumery. Lavender oil is obtained from the plant by three methods, all of them still in use today:

1. Direct distillation - also known as "direct fire distillation": This is the oldest form of distillation; though technically refined it has essentially remained unchanged. In direct distillation the plant material is thrown into a cauldron filled with water which is then heated over an open fire (hence its name), until the water starts boiling. This process needs to be handled very carefully, because even the slightest overheating may "burn" the essence which will then smell accordingly. Yet for some plants, like rose and orange flowers, direct distillation is the only possibility. We may compare direct distillation to the boiling of vegetables in a pot.

2. Steam distillation: Even today this is the most widely applied method of distillation, used for many different plants. The illustration on the previous page explains the process of steam distillation. The lower part of the still is filled with water over which a metal grid is placed. Plant material is pressed tightly against this grid until the still is fully loaded. The water is heated; the rising low pressure steam passes through the plant material and releases the essential oils. We can compare this method to the steaming of vegetables.

3. High Pressure steam distillation: Here water and plant material are kept in separate containers. The water is heated, extremely hot steam emerges from a pipe and passes, under high pressure, through the plant material. Today high pressure distil-

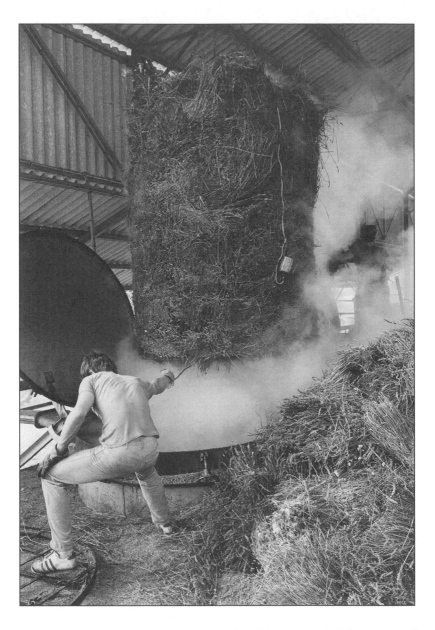

After distillation is completed, plant material is removed from still and can be processed further for many different purposes

lation is the preferred method for the production of lavender oil.

It allows a high yield of an essential oil rich in ester and is much faster than any other form of distillation. We can compare high pressure steam distillation to the boiling of vegetables in a pressure cooker.

All three methods, however, lead to the same conclusion: steam, together with the vapour of released essences, is gathered into a steadily narrowing pipe (the so-called "goose-neck") which passes through a condensor; they cool down and leave the condensor in the form of water and the essential oil which are then collected together in a container known as a Florentine vase. The lavender oil lies on the surface of the water and is siphoned into a separate container.

A number of factors determine how much essence can be obtained from lavender plants: age, weather, cultivation and the amount of time between the harvest and the actual processing of the plants. Four to seven year old plants give the highest yield. High temperatures in June and July guarantee a higher yield; cold spells are counter-productive. Cultivated lavender yields more lavender oil than lavender growing in the wild. Lavender has to be processed within 48 hours after cutting to avoid a lower yield of essence.

The Fine Art of Distillation

The distillation of lavender is an art almost as complex as alchemy was considered to be in ancient times. Close and relentless attention, technical skills and much experience are needed. In addition, the distiller has constantly to question his own priorities: does he want quantity or does he want quality?

Often essential oils are characterized as "spirits", the "soul" of a plant, and the process of distillation is designed to separate these "subtle" and "psychic" essences from the "coarse" and "material". The way in which we achieve this goal largely determines the quality of the oil we shall receive as the end product. Of course, high temperatures and high steam pressure will grant a higher yield. However, to use them means to use force - a force that interferes with the complex composition of an essential oil. Such methods degrade its quality.

Until now lavender oil has been found to be composed of 170 components, some of them rather delicate and sensitive to pressure and heat, both of which will annihilate them if used excessively and forcefully. Since the spectrum of operation of an essence depends solely on the completeness of its components, loss of components means loss of quality.

The process of distillation could be divided into two stages: after two thirds of its duration 90% of the components have been released, but it takes as much as one more third of the duration to obtain the remaining 10%. For reasons of economy distillation is often prematurely halted resulting in either the lack of certain components and/or considerably altering the ratio of the different components within the oil.

This may actually be a rather productive approach to be pursued in perfumery: by eliminating components or changing their ratios within the oil, manipulation of distillation procedures will yield interesting new fragrances. However, in aromatherapy, we need lavender oil containing all of its components to allow for its full spectrum of operation. We need an essence that has been obtained as slowly and gently as is conducive to the completeness of its components.

Pure lavender oil should be as satisfying to our nose as a well orchestrated piece of music is to our ears. It should consist of a melodious basic theme, paraphrased by different instruments in different keys that all blend together - a composition in the true sense of the word.

Lavender is Not All the Same -
The Different Varieties

Lavender:	*lavendula angustifolia*
Synonyms:	*lavendula officinalis / Lavendula Vera*
Colour:	blue/purple flowers
Height:	60 cm (approx. 2ft)
Odour:	fine and sweet with no camphor
Use:	important ingredient in high class perfumes
Yield:	0.5 to 1.5% essential oil
Dissemination:	in the wild it grows at high altitudes; indigenous to France.
Flowering Period:	early July - early August
Main Ingredients:	linalyl acetate and linalool

Mr Denny of Bridestone says: "This is a dwarf shrub offering a relatively small yield of oil which is entirely free from camphor". Its natural habitat is between 1000 and 2000 meters altitude in the French Sea Alps. The best qualities grow above 1200 meters (3600ft) altitude, and are sometimes called "Mont Blanc". The flowers of wild growing lavender come in many colours, white, pink and purple blossoms often appearing on the same plant. However, the colour of the flowers has no bearing on the quality of the oil; at least we don't know of any such correlation. But we do know that aromatherapists prefer the oil of wild growing lavender to any other lavender oil.

Spike Lavender:	*lavendula latifolia*
Colour:	greyish flowers
Height:	80 to 90 cm (approx. 3ft)
Odour:	camphoraceous

Use:	soap, lower priced toiletries and washing powders
Yield:	0.5 to 1.0% essential oil
Dissemination:	grows at lower altitudes, mainly between 200 and 500 meters above sea level in Spain, France and Yugosla via; indigenous to Spain.
Main Ingredients:	Cineole and camphor

Mr Denny says: "This is a strong growing shrub giving a fairly large yield of oil which smells strongly of camphor. It occurs naturally at lower altitudes around the northern Mediterranean shore, especially in Spain". Because of its high content of camphor, aromatherapists like to use it to treat ailments of the bronchial tubes.

Lavandin:	*lavendula intermedia / hybridia* (the hybrid of true lavender and spike lavender)
Colour:	varies through all shades of blue, to pink and even white
Height:	varies between 40 and 100 cm (up to over 3ft)
Use:	widely in perfumery
Yield:	1.5 to 2.5% essential oil
Altitude:	up to 500 meters (1500ft) above sea level

Flowering period: July - August

Main ingredients: due to its hybrid nature the composition of its essential oil is much more variable than either of its parents. This hybrid originated through spontaneous pollination by insects of *Lavendula angustifolia* and *Lavendula latifolia* at altitudes of 500 meters (1500ft) where both varieties grow in the wild, and for this very reason even lavender grown in cultivation may contain some lavandin. At higher altitudes hybrids don't form.

Mr Denny says: "As commonly occurs with this type of cross,

the hybrid is sterile but stronger than either of its parents. It provides very large yields of camphoraceous oil".

How We Can Determine the Purity of an Essence

Unfortunately, because it is lower priced, lavandin is used to "cut" lavender oil. Since lavandin is itself a natural essence and different mainly in terms of its lower content of ester, this adulteration is not easy to prove. Sometimes more ester is added. This, however, only constitutes a further falsification of the natural essence.

The quotas of lavender are limited. For example, the naturally restricted area for cultivation in England allows for only a certain amount of English lavender oil. Consequently, on occasion, French oils have been proclaimed as "English Oils", whereas so-called "French Oils" were actually produced in Italy or Spain.

Spectography, chromatographic analysis and "alternative" methods like Kirilian photography are used to test the quality of a supposedly "natural" essence. Since there are numerous ways to falsify an essence, it is not always easy to track them down. Essential oils are highly prized natural materials, sold in large quantities. For the sake of additional profit, "business minded" growers may therefore be tempted to tamper with them. As in any other competitive industry, perfumery has not always been completely honest. Thus, direct and personal contact with the actual grower, a relationship of mutual trust that has stood the test of time, may be a better protection against fraud than any scientific analysis, however sophisticated in itself it may be. Also, consumers have become more informed in recent years. This, together with the growing demand of aromatherapists for absolutely pure essences, has contributed to a shift in attitude.

The countries producing essential oils try to safeguard their reputation with tighter quality controls and by issuing clearly defined marks of origin, a development which can only be welcomed.

Besides chemical and physical analysis and good relations with the actual producer, one other method should help to protect us against being sold oils that have been adulterated: a keen sense of smell. Such a well-trained sense of smell may only develop over years of experience. Once gained, however, it will never betray us.

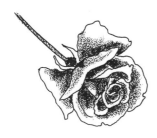

Where and How
Lavender Is Cultivated

No country has a more intimate relationship with lavender than France, still the most important producer of lavender oil in the world. Lavender thrives on the chalky soils, in the dry ravines and hot summers of Haute Provence. But the demand for lavender is constantly growing, even today, and France alone cannot satisfy that demand. Thus lavender is also cultivated successfully in other regions of Europe and in many parts of the world.

France

Lavender is the soul of Haute-Provence.
Jean Giono

As the nineteenth century ended, the "Golden Age" of perfumery dawned. All of a sudden the demand for lavender rose significantly, in other countries as much as in France itself. Consequently, in the traditional lavender growing areas of France, the picking of lavender changed from an occasional activity to an organized commercial venture.

Only one or two decades earlier a considerable rural exodus had depleted the French Sea Alps of a substantial part of their population. Chalky soils, harsh cold winters and almost rainless hot summers had made agriculture in higher elevations a thankless task that offered few if any rewards. The industrial revolu-

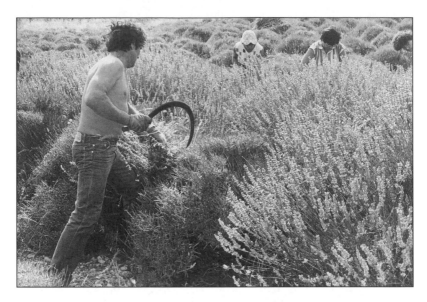

Picking lavender by hand in Haute Provence

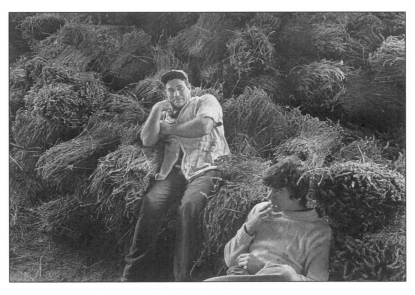

Two French pickers after harvesting

tion first lured the men and then whole families into the cities farther north. Land that had been arable for centuries was now deserted, and only hardy, easily satisfied plants could survive on those deserted fields. Foremost among them was lavender (above 600m or 1200ft above sea level) and lavendin (between 500m and 600m or 1500 and 1800ft above sea level). Women, children and herdsmen picked this wild growing lavender, selling it to the expanding perfumery industry at Grasse which was endeavouring to keep pace with events. The growing population in the cities of Europe and the fashion of the times constantly added to the demand for more and more fragrant substances. Bringing, as it did, a new economic independence, this development turned out to be a blessing for the pickers and small distilleries of the region. Finally they had found a crop that was much in demand, and moreover, more durable than any vegetable or grain. Much had changed for the traditionally poor people dwelling between Mont Ventoux and the gorges of Verdon.

In 1920, 100 tons of lavender were distilled (90% true lavender and 10% spike). But the days of the predominance of wild growing lavender were numbered. Increasingly lavandin was grown systematically in fields much like any other culti-vated crop. Its astounding rise to prominence started in 1924 with the distillate of 1 ton of lavandin; the annual yield peaked at 1000 tons and has only recently begun to diminish.

Lavandin, cloned lavender that could more easily satisfy the growing demand for lavender oil because of higher yield, was mass cultivated. So much cheaper to produce than true lavender, it furthermore fulfilled the demand for mass produced scented soaps, toilet waters and perfumes, now used by almost every-body instead of just the chosen few of the upper classes.

In today's France Lavandin still covers more acres than any other kind of lavender. Many varieties have been tested since the boom began in the 1930s: lavandin abrialis, lavandin super, "Maillette", and "Grosso" (the last two bearing the names of their cultivators), to mention just a few. The overall goal of this process of selection has been hardiness, longevity, optimum yield, and, in some instances, more intensely coloured flowers. However, by propagation through cuttings, the grower ends up with varieties of lavandin which are identical because they originate from the same source.

In this respect true, wild growing lavender, is the very opposite. Every plant is unique, a personality of its own. So unique in fact, that its flowers, may come in many different shades of colour, and even yield several lavender oils that differ significantly in terms of the ratio of their components. Wild growing lavender plants are thus "individuals", not laboratory products" or "clones".

Recently, market forces seem to have shifted the interest in the French lavender industry again, and this time in the opposite direction. The demand for true lavender is rising, whereas the demand for lavandin is in decline. The growers accommodate the shift by trying out new varieties from different origins and elevations and protecting them through special designations (very much like the French wine industry and their *appellations controllées*). Independent inspection agencies test the oils for quality and purity, giving out certificates which inform the buyer about the exact source of his oil. There are even strictly organically-grown varieties available. Without exception they are either obtained from wild growing plants or from smaller farms that are located in higher altitudes.

But history and facts do not give us the whole picture. To really appreciate what lavender means for Haute Provence we should experience the plant in its natural habitat:

"I spent the whole summer backpacking in Southern France. I hiked over the high plateaux of Western Provence, followed brittle, chalky deer paths that almost gleamed like the white sun in midday. Step after step, day after day, and always a sea of purple flowers at my feet, filling the land, touching the horizon, while overarching blue was the dome above my head. From dawn to dusk, bees were humming, assiduously going about

their chores. Some of the dwarf-like lavender plants reminded me, strangely enough, of sea urchins, but their fragrance first filled my nose, then my heart with stillness, peace - exhilarating confidence... All this, all these memories are now contained in one small bottle... of lavender oil on my desk".

Jean Giono

England

Mitcham, in the county of Surrey, used to be the main lavender producing region in England in the 1800s, with "Mitcham-Lavender" gaining international acclaim. However, Mitcham and its surrounding districts soon attracted London business-men who wanted to live in the tranquil atmosphere, and slowly it became part of what is now called the "stockbroker belt". Lavender production ceased in Mitcham when landowners found that "growing houses" was more profitable than growing lavender.

Lavender was also grown commercially by the Ransome family in Hitchin, a town to the North of London in the county of Hertfordshire. A business, still in existence today, known as "William Ransome", was started in 1846 to supply lavender oil to perfume and cosmetic houses. The business moved a little further north to Cambridgeshire, where, to this day, a herb farm grows medicinal herbs, and several acres of lavender. The company still boasts a Ransome on its payroll, a great grandson of the original founder. The farm is a commercial business and is not open to visitors at any time.

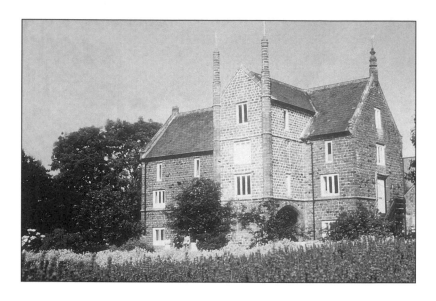

Lavender field in Norfolk

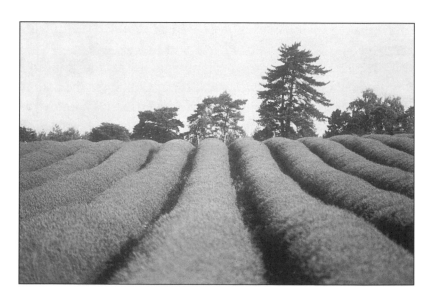

Rows of lavender in Norfolk

Norfolk Lavender

Norfolk Lavender, I feel, deserves a separate section, even though it technically comes under "England".

Norfolk Lavender was started in the 1930s as the result of one man's dream. Having witnessed the demise of lavender in Mitcham, Linneaus Chilvers planned to resurrect the English lavender industry. As lavender is a hardy plant which likes light, well-drained, fairly alkaline soil, Linn Chilvers felt that north Norfolk, with its lower than average rainfall, would be an ideal place for lavender to grow. Much experimentation with different species of lavender was necessary and many years were devoted to the search for a disease resistant plant which would produce a good quality oil in sufficient quantities to make the project a success. Developing a lavender farm is a long and complicated business. To illustrate this further, let us quote from the booklet The Story of Norfolk Lavender:

"When developing new hybrids from seeds, it is necessary first to select an individual bush, and to distil the flowers from that bush alone in order to obtain its oil, which must then be tested for its perfume note, chemical compound, and indicated yield. If all of these are satisfactory, then, in October of the same year, the cuttings can be taken which will provide enough plants for a quantitive assessment about five years later. If that is successful, cuttings can be taken from those plants for planting on a field-scale. As the field will not be in full bearing for at least another five years, the span from choosing a likely plant to harvesting an acre or so of its oil cannot be less than ten years".

1932 saw the origin of Norfolk lavender when Linneaus Chilvers went into partnership with Francis Dusgate and planted six acres of land (33,000 rooted cuttings). The present lavender farm consists of six varieties which were chosen from nearly 100 hybrids.

Initially there was no distillery on site, and the lavender crop was sent away for distillation. But its high quality soon attracted the attention of Yardleys, so that in 1936, two copper stills were brought over from France. The success of Norfolk Lavender meant that more land was needed, and in later years 50 acres of the Sandringham Estate (one of the homes of Queen Elizabeth II) was made available to Norfolk Lavender.

Originally the lavender was harvested by hand using a small curved sickle. The women would place the cut lavender into tubs, which would be taken to a forewoman. A token would be handed out for each full tub, and at the end of the day these tokens were exchanged for money.

When harvesting by hand became uneconomical, it was necessary to replant the fields so that a mechanical harvester could be used. In 1955, replanting was in rows, with six feet between each row, and a harvester was designed. The harvested cuts and prunes the lavender hedge in one operation, and a conveyor belt transports the cut material into sacks, which are tied and put into piles to await collection. These sacks, after loading, are taken back to Caley Mill where the process of unloading and distillation is carried out.

Fortunate visitors to Caley Mill, in July and August, can witness the entire operation, from the unloading of the sacks, to loading up the stills, treading down the plant material, and finally the emergence of the essential oil and water from the Florentine, amid a continuous flow of cold steam. The air is heavy with the scent of lavender, and it is easy to feel transported to an earlier time and a different pace of life.

The Jersey Lavender Farm

The grandparents of David Christie bought some land in Jersey in 1919. It was duneland, and nothing much grew there, but over the years some trees were planted and a home was built.

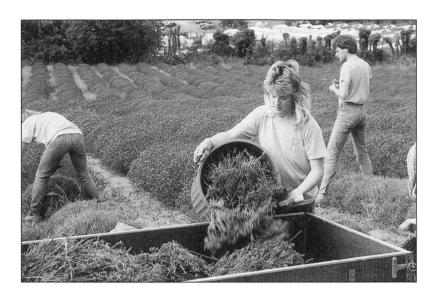

The small growing Jersey lavender is cut and loaded onto a cart

The next generation divided up the land and David and Elizabeth Christie inherited 10-12 acres of sandy dunes. It was difficult to know what to grow there, and they thought about carrots and then asparagus.

At this time David was a school teacher in Winchester and during his studies had come across an article about Norfolk Lavender. He also recalled that his grandmother's lavender hedge had thrived perfectly well over the years, and set about costing the viability of planting lavender. David bought 25,000 young plants and the first two thirds of the existing farm was planted in 1983, the remainder in 1984. Three varieties of lavender were chosen to give a continuous harvest from mid-June to mid-August. 6.5 acres are currently under production, and the farm boasts an impressive collection of 160 growing herbs.

The harvesting is carried out by hand; the cut lavender is placed in drums and taken to the still where it is distilled each day. It is a small, family run business, and visitors are made welcome. 90% of the crop id distilled, and the remaining 10% is dried for herb sachets.

Three years after planting the farm opened its doors to visitors, and now, a further seven years on, the lavender crop has yielded more than ever before. The visitors are increasing, and the desolate sandy acres have been transformed into a healthy, viable enterprise, proving that the only thing to match the tenacity of lavender's growth in adverse conditions is man's determination to make his vision into a reality.

Japan

Lavender is also grown on Hokkaido, the most northerly of the four main islands that make up Japan. The soil appears to be predominantly sandy, and the climate, being on the latitude of 42-45 degrees north of the equator, would be similar to that of the *Alpes Maritimes* in Southern France.

In Hokkaido, lavender is cultivated for its beautiful deep purple bloom, and the stems are hand cut to a uniform length. Drying is done naturally, without any artificial heat, and is carried out by taking small bunches of lavender, binding the stems, and then suspending the bunches from taut horizontal ropes. In this way, the closely hung branches of lavender form a ceiling of purple, and the flowers are preserved in perfect condition. The lavender crop is grown for its flowers and not for its essential oil.

Tasmania

In the early 1920s Mr and Mrs Denny, with hope in their hearts and a bag of lavender seeds from the French Alps, left England for a new life in Tasmania to grow true lavender - *lavendula angustifolia*. By the summer of 1924 a quarter of an acre field in North Lilydale had yielded enough flowers for a distillation. This being completed, the oil was sent to London for appraisal by experts who declared it completely free of camphor.

Over the next few decades, more and more land was planted with *Lavendula angustifolia* and a distillery was built in 1930. The first exports of lavender oil were in 1935. In 1946, after many ups and downs with the growing lavender farm, the two sons of the family joined their father and set about the expansion of the industry. In 1948 further land, near Nabowla, Tasmania, was planted with lavender cuttings. Then in 1949, a plant selection programme was started to pinpoint the genotype which would have the best qualities. For just as brothers and sisters differ in appearance, although from the same parents, so too do the lavender plants which are grown from seeds of the parent plant. What was being sought was a plant with natural vigour, good oil quality, and high yields together with long life. Hundreds of genotypes were tested over a period of eleven years, and at one time these trials covered nearly 100 acres. As a result of these tests thirteen strains were selected which had all of the desired characteristics.

These plants were the parents of the Tasmanian lavender industry. It took many years to restock the plantations with the selected cuttings. This selection process also allowed the Denny family to combine the early, mid-season and late flowering types, so ensuring a continuous harvest throughout the month of January. Although this programme of testing must appear slow and tedious, the results showed that the lavender plants were able to produce three times the oil yield of the unselected plantations. So, the selected fields yielded sixty instead of twenty kilos per hectare (a hectare is 2.471 acres).

The Bridestowe Estate has developed phenomenally well during the past sixty or so years, but there are still two important areas which are under investigation. One is the control of fungi, which may be transferred from old tree roots in the ground. The

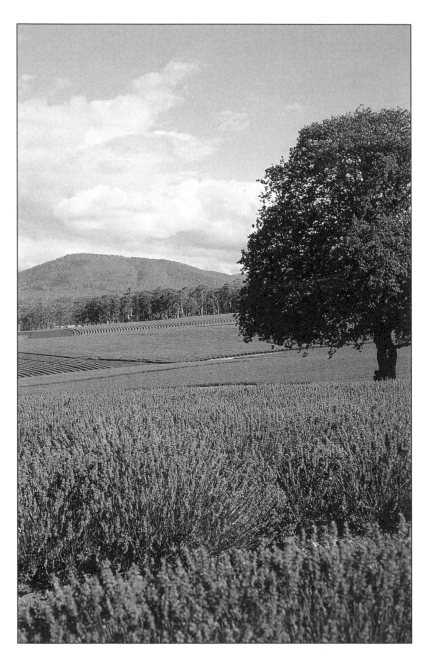

Lavender fields in Tasmania

other is the havoc caused by the weather, as the crop is still susceptible to frost damage after the flower buds have been formed.

Even though lavender is a deep rooted plant and can survive in very dry weather, a lack of rain can sometimes interfere with the yield. However, this never accounts for more than 12% of the crop, and it is not economically viable to irrigate land covering more than 150 acres.

The harvesting, which used to be carried out by hand, needed to be mechanised. The present harvester, which was developed by the company, can cut and pack 2.5 tons of flowers per hour, ready for distillation. It would require more than ninety men to compete with that rate of harvesting. Only 15% of the Australian lavender yield is sold within the country; the rest is exported to the Americas and Europe.

Lavender Around The Globe

While writing about the international lavender situation, I plotted the locations on the map and was surprised to see the pattern that emerged on a global scale.

On a latitude of 40-45 degrees north lie the lavender farms in Hokkaido, Japan. On the same latitude lie the French Sea Alps. Then, if we look south of the equator to latitude 40-45 degrees, we have Tasmania.

Does this mean that the huge part of North America which lies on this latitude could be growing lavender? I think this is a distinct possibility, as lavender once grew in Washington State and California.

If we were to take a globe and draw a lavender coloured line around it at latitude 40-45 north, we have the Soviet Union which produces lavender oil in its southern districts and on the Crimean Peninsula, Hungary which produces lavender oil in Tihany, northern Italy and Southern France where lavender grows in the Sea Alps and North America where lavender was once cultivated in Washington and California. Taking our imaginary lavender line to be real, we would have a line of lavender plantations stretching from Boston on the east coast to Northern California on the west coast. Apart from Australia and South America, there is little landmass at 40-45 south, but we could expect lavender to grow in New Zealand on either side of the Cook Strait. And in South America the lavender line would cut across Argentina where lavender was once grown in the highland of Mendoza to midway between Buenos Aires and the southernmost tip. The Jersey lavender is on a slightly more northerly latitude, around 50 degrees, with Norfolk Lavender (at around 52 degrees) being the most northerly location.

It is my opinion that there is not enough lavender grown on a worldwide scale, given its versatility and safeness in use together with its ability to grow where little else will. These factors make it a perfect candidate for further development as a product that would benefit mankind. In this multi-coloured world we need a little more lavender.

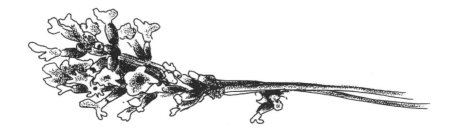

Lavender:
Facts and Figures

This chapter is about the chemical analysis of lavender. I used to think this aspect of aromatherapy was boring and of no interest to me, so I avoided it. However, the deeper my relationship with essential oils becomes, the more I want to understand how they work. And the more I found out about the complex chemical structures, the more respectful I am of the plants, their oils and the Creator of the plant kingdom.

Can you imagine the creation of just one odoriferous molecule? With its structures of carbon atoms, hydrogen atoms and oxygen atoms, all of which enable us to smell it, to recognize it so that eventually we can give it a name like "linalyl acetate". Then can you imagine repeating the procedure, only this time changing the arrangement of the atoms, giving it a slightly different smell, so that we can give it another name like "linalool". And then imagine that you keep on inventing more and more odoriferous molecules and arranging them so that they each have a distinctive smell and look. Finally, blend them together to create the aroma that we recognise as "lavender". What an incredible perfumer! What an incredible scientist! And then imagine giving this beautiful perfume so many healing qualities. What an incredible doctor! What an amazing healer!

For many centuries man has been intrigued by this fascinating and complex botanical, but only in the nineteenth century did he finally begin to analyse it in any detail. In 1818 hydrocarbons containing terpenes were found to consist regularly of five carbon and eight hydrogen atoms. In 1925 Boulet discovered Courmarine. Now that scientists and technicians have developed very sophisticated analytical machines, we are able to look at the composition of the oil and ascertain its chemical breakdown.

Many books have been published and many articles have been written on the scientific research into essential oils. The most notable English language author in this field was Ernest Guenther whose work "The Essential Oils" was published in sixteen volumes in 1952. In Germany, Eduard Gildemeister came up with a similar achievement. His *Ätherische Öle* originally came out in 1899 and was updated in the 1920s and again in 1956. Since then the technological advances in analytical research have enabled even more constituents to be identified. The most recent findings are those of Dr Brian Lawrence. Here is a summary of his analysis of lavender oil:

"Almost half the constituents are **Esters:**
linalyl acetate
lavandulyl acetate
geranyl acetate
terpenyl acetate
hexenyl acetate

the next largest chemical group are the
Terpene Alcohols
linalool
terpinen 4 ol
alpha terpineol
borneol
geraniol

then, in smaller quantities, we have **Terpenes**
pinene
myorene
carene
limonene
ocimene

and then the **Aldehydes**
benzaldehyde
hexanal
citral
cuminaldehyde

and finally the **Ketones**
methylheptone
camphor".

However, as we have said before, there is no such thing as the one and only "correct lavender essence". Among the many factors influencing the ratio of its components are: variety, place of cultivation, weather, time of harvest, type and duration of distillation and so forth. To illustrate how different high quality essences may be the chart below shows variations of ratio of the chemical compounds of both French lavender and lavender flower oil obtained by steam distillation:

	lavender oil	lavender flower oil
linalyl acetate (linaly butyrate,	30-35%	35-50%
geranly acetate)	35-50%	35-50%
linalool (geranoil, nerol)	0.5-0.8%	3.5%
courmarine	0%	5%
umbeiliferon methyl ether	6%	5%
terpenes (pinene) cineole	traces	traces
ethylmylketone	traces	traces
caproic acid geranly capronate	traces	traces
bornyl acetate (acetic acid)		

from Paul Jellinek: *Die psychologischen Grundlagen der Parfümerie* (The Psycological Basics of Perfurmery), Heidelberg, 1965

Scientific Proof for the Healing Powers of Lavender

Although aromatherapy did not come out of nowhere and has developed over centuries rather than decades, scientific analysis of the plants and essences only started in the late nineteenth century. However, there has been more and more research in recent years. We still cannot describe with absolute certainty how essential oils promote healing, but we know more than we have ever known about this process. We therefore want to share with you some of the insights into the working of lavender oil that science has revealed thus far.

In his *History of Scent* Roy Genders writes: "In the early nineteenth century at the Pasteur Institute, Professor Omelt-Schenki proved that the typhoid bacillus was destroyed within forty-five minutes in the air containing the vapour of the oil of cinnamon and that tuberculosis bacilli were destroyed within twelve hours of exposure to the vapour of oil of lavender".

In the mid-nineteenth century it was noticed that people in the flower-growing districts of Southern France hardly ever suffered from tuberculosis, whilst in the rest of France tuberculosis was rampant. Closer examination revealed that the workers were also free from other respiratory diseases, and the assumption that the essential oils in the plants were responsible for their good health led, in 1887, to the first recorded laboratory tests to prove that essential oils had anti-bacterial properties.

In the next few years many essential oils were tested on microorganisms, and lavender was one of the essences shown to be most effective in combatting yellow fever. Yet, such discoveries did not promote success. Sagarin concludes: "...it seems very strange that, the more tests that were done on essential oils the less they were acknowledged and put to use by the medical doctors".

Since then much testing and research by means of both laboratory tests and clinical trials have been undertaken to prove the therapeutic properties of essential oils. In his *Modern Pharmacognosy* of 1959 Egil Ramstad says: "In general, essential oils are antiseptic and bactericidal; they have been used since antiquity as preservatives and are also used today as germicides and fungicides". He gives a table of oils together with the concentration needed to prevent bacteria from developing in meat broth and claims that 3-4 mls of lavender oil in one litre of meat broth would inhibit the growth of bacteria.

Professor Paolo Rovesti at Milan University has been researching the therapeutic uses of essential oils for many years and has written numerous books on his findings. He points out that the pleasantly smelling essential oils are more acceptable and more effective for people suffering from nervous tension. Lavender is named as one of the most useful essences for relieving anxiety. "Very conclusive experiments have been carried out in various clinics for nervous diseases, on patients affected by hysteria or psychic depression".

Recent research carried out at Warwick University backs up Rovesti's statement, as Steve van Toller, working with very sophisticated brain scanning computers, concludes: "...the brain simply rejects odours perceived as unpleasant." It therefore seems logical that odours which are perceived as pleasant would have more chance of bringing about a therapeutic change, because the brain has accepted them, and allowed them to reach the limbic system, a group of brain structures at the inner border of the cerebral hemispheres that include neurons involved in emotions. In states of extreme fear or anger the limbic system can be influential enough to dominate activity in other parts of the brain.

Professor Torii, from Toho University in Japan, has been conducting experiments with essential oils in order to measure objectively, the psychological effects of odours on brain activity. Odours chosen for tests were those which were known to be sedative or stimulating, notably jasmine and lavender.

Here is a brief summary of his findings: "There is an electrical phenomena in the human brain that is called 'Contingent Negative Variation (CNV)'. This is an upward shift in the brain waves recorded by electrodes attached to the scalp, occurring in situations where subjects are expecting something to happen. For example, a subject is given a sound stimulus followed by a light stimulus. When the light appears, subjects are requested to turn it off as quickly as possible. Within the interval between the two stimuli (the expectancy period) there appears a slow upward shift from the baseline of the subject's electroencephalogram (EEG). This shift in the EEG is what is called 'Contingent

Negative Variation (CNV)'... In our study we examined whether CNV can be used objectively to observe stimulating and sedative effects of odours. Our experiments showed that the odour of jasmine, which is said to have a stimulating effect, increased CNV amplitude, while the fragrance of lavender, which is said to have a sedative effect, decreased our subjects' CNV... We were able to prove scientifically the truth of the old adage that jasmine stimulates and lavender relaxes."

Lavender in Modern Aromatherapy

We have mentioned already that René-Maurice Gattefossé coined the term "aromatherapy" in 1928 and that, inspired by one striking personal experience, he devoted the remainder of his life to essential oil research. Among his many students, Jean Valnet and Marguerite Maury deserve to be mentioned because of their own pioneering work. But countless other individuals have contributed to the development of aromatherapy which has only received the attention it rightfully deserves in recent years.

Throughout the world essences are tested scientifically and the properties traditionally attributed to them are found, to a large extent, to be close to the truth. There is nothing wrong with this, because facts and figures will eventually convince us of the value of gentle modes of healing and preventive medicine such as aromatherapy.

How the Aromatherapists Treat Their Clients With Lavender Oil

Lavender oil is one of the most renowned essences. It is also the most widely used. Since essential oils represent highly concentrated plant substances, aromatherapy could be considered a kind of "nuclear" phytotherapy.

As we can see from the tables above, the chemical compounds of lavender oil are known by now. We thus should be in a

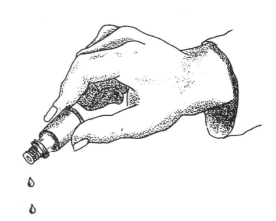

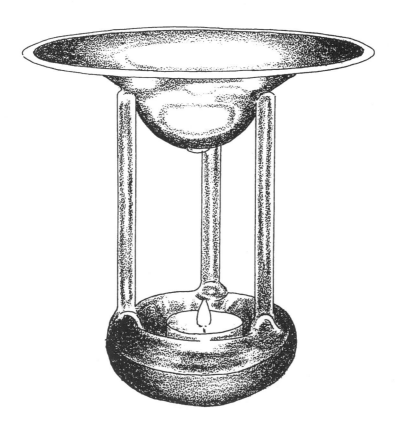

position to produce them synthetically, ...but still would fail. Though we actually can reproduce and mix the "parts", the "whole" eludes us, because our artificial composition does not work in the same ways the original oil does. Synthetic essences may actually be harmful, as we can see from a case history that Dr Valnet describes in his book on aromatherapy. He had started to treat a patient suffering from anal fistula with pure lavender oil, apparently with some success, when the patient had to leave for a trip. Unfortunately, the patient forgot to take his own lavender oil with him, and was forced to substitute it with some other lavender oil that he purchased in a local pharmacy. Its use resulted in outright disaster. The fistula became inflamed, he suffered from intense pain, and could not sit for two entire weeks. The "lavender oil" he had purchased had not been 100% pure and natural and he had had to endure the dire consequences. This story serves as an instructive example, reminding us to insist on good quality lavender oil, for our personal and professional use. The life force and healing powers of natural essences thus far remain prerogative of nature and cannot be copied synthetically.

Robert Tisserand describes lavender as the most versatile and useful of all essential oils. It stimulates the growth of healthy new skin and accelerates the healing of damaged skin. It expedites the formation of healthy new cells and, in this regard, we could rightfully describe it as promoting rejuvenation. Furthermore it stimulates the formation and activity of a certain type of healthy white blood cell (and thus would never trigger leukaemia).

Most books on lavender agree on the medicinal properties of its essential oil being:

antispasmodic
analgesic
sedative (when normal doses have been applied)
stimulating (when higher doses have been applied)
antidepressive
antiseptic

carminative
cicatrizant
diuretic
sudorific
cardiotonic

Main indications are:
spasms
irritability
insomnia
infectious diseases
respiratory ailments (asthma, spasmodic coughs, whooping
coughs, influenza, bronchitis)
melancholia (anxiety, general physical and mental
debility)
neurasthenia
neuralgic pains
swoons
tension
myalgia (muscular pain)
menstrual pains and cramps
oliguria (insufficient flow of urine)
hypertension
leucorrhoea
headaches
migraine
vertigo
cystitis
alopecia (loss of hair)
halitosis (bad breath)
otalgia (ear aches)
wounds and sores of all descriptions (simple, atonic,
infected, gangrenous, syphilitic, chancres, anal fistula)
burns
eczema
acne and acne rosacea

anxiety
depression
herpes
insect bites
general skin care

Aromatherapy in France

In France, aromatherapy is practised mainly by medical doctors, and in a very particular way. Essential oils are given orally to combat infections of the body such as urinary problems, genital diseases, and bronchial and other afflictions of the lungs.

In order for the doctors to decide upon the correct essence or blend of essences to be used, they first of all establish a so-called "aromatagram". A swab is taken from the site of infection and cultured in a Petri dish. The culture is then divided into several sterile dishes; drops of different essential oils are added to each dish and left for several hours. The essential oils which have killed off the bacteria in the cultures are the oils which are prescribed for the patient. The patient then takes the prescription to a pharmacy where it is made up by the pharmacist. Doctors are prohibited by French law from dispensing the oils themselves.

The medical profession in France takes aromatherapy very seriously indeed. Medical aromatherapy is taught at a post-graduate level in several medical colleges in France. The first university "chair" in alternative medicine was that of phytotherapy at the Universite de Paris Nord. The Professor is Dr Paul Belaiche who also runs a surgery and has a very high success rate with his patients. He first uses the aromatagram to find the essential oils which will work most effectively against fungi, bacteria, and viruses. Lavender oil is very often one of the essences prescribed.

Some Examples of the Practice of Aromatherapy in England

Hospitals all over the British Isles are now using essential oils with remarkable results. Ros Wise of the John Radcliffe Hospital in Oxford reports: "At the Churchill Hospital in Oxford, sister Helen Passant has been using aromatherapy for many years to care for the elderly on a long-stay ward". Also incorporated are music, natural juices, massage and meditation. "Through rhythm, touch and fragrance, the ward is transformed into a home - a place of comfort and warmth from which to pass eventually into another world".

Ros Wise herself works in the John Radcliffe Hospital, in a general and vascular ward. "We practice primary nursing, which gave us the freedom and encouragement to include aromatherapy in our care plans, and the continuity necessary to monitor results". Lavender is used in the wards to help induce sleep and a restful state; it is also used to purify the air, thereby bringing to bear its prophylactic properties. "Since our initial steps with aromatherapy, we are daily discovering new areas in which the essential oils meet the needs of our patients. We use them as a complement to orthodox treatment and care". Pre-operative patients are given lavender and geranium baths to sooth anxiety.

Lavender oil vapour has proved effective in the relief of migraine. "Unable to take her usual medication after surgery, one long-term migraine sufferer was willing to try the lavender oil. She was surprised to find that gradually, over a period of about an hour, her migraine lifted". The fragrances of the essential oils"... take the patient away from the hospital ward and the sick role in which he or she may feel so helpless... For the surgical patient, it is myfirm belief that aromatherapy helps to take the anxiety out of being in a hospital, and quickens the patient's return to selfcare", and Sister Passant of the Churchill Hospital adds with pride: "We no longer use any sedatives on our ward at night".

In the Beeson Ward of the Radcliffe Infirmary, Oxford, the Nurse Practitioners in the Oxford Nursing Development Unit are using a selection of essential oils, but mainly lavender. As well as for its sedative properties, lavender essence is applied to combat pain. "We also use the oils, mainly lavender again, to enhance analgesia... we had a man who had a lot of pain before his amputation, and after the amputation he had a lot of phantom limb pain... this was an amputation below the knee, so one of the nurses massaged the upper part of the leg. This brought about almost complete pain relief for ninety minutes after the massage, which was done with diluted lavender oil".

The Oxford Nursing Development Unit is something of an experiment, as patients are put under the care of "nurse practitioners". The most striking feature about the ward is that patients are told why they are in hospital, what exactly is wrong with them and then given the choice of opting for aromatherapy massage or accepting the conventional sedatives.

The approach to patients is a holistic one, and they are cared for as individuals, rather than merely having their medical problems taken care of.

The latest UK hospital to incorporate the use of lavender oil into the patient's daily routine, is a maternity hospital just north of London. The Ward Sister, having seen how lavender healed the perineum of those mothers taking lavender baths after childbirth, has obtained the approval of the hospital consultants, and is undertaking a full clinical trial on the beneficial action of lavender oil.

Aromatherapy in Germany

Not contenting themselves with commonly accepted approaches, aromatherapists in Germany are increasingly focusing on the subtle, vibrational effects of the oils. Each oil has unique qualities and can be applied for certain purposes (for example as antiseptic or antispasmodic) which in turn define its "personality". Likewise, when first trying aromatherapy, every client brings with him or herself, typical problems and unique characteristics. It is therefore important for the aromatherapist to find the essences most fitting for each client, for only these essences will eventually support a healthy change, accommodating physical, emotional, and mental balance. The better an essence agrees with the physical and psychological make-up of a client the better the chances are of genuine healing.

Martin Henglein of Munich has developed a special olfactory test: the patient briefly smells four essential oils, which relate to four areas basic to human existence and activity. Afterwards he or she is encouraged to describe spontaneously whatever images and associations come to mind, stimulated by the aroma of these four oils. Negative associations, in the worst case the rejection of an oil, point to a likely problem in the area related to this particular essence. The client's first spontaneous descriptions determine which oils are going to be used in a treatment consisting mainly of inhalation and/ or application to certain acupuncture points.

The four essences used in the first olfactory test are: rosemary, bergamot, geranium and patchouli. In the context of Martin Henglein's test, rosemary represents the centre of our existence - the "I", self-assertion, a healthy degree of forcefulness and aggression. Bergamot represents our connection to the mental planes, our ability to communicate, as well as mobility, flexibility and nimbleness. Geranium represents our openness to other people, our ability for normal and nourishing emotional involvement and our sensibility to respond to the peculiarities and needs of another person. Patchouli represents the ability to trust our bodies as well as "joyous acceptance" of whatever we may encounter - it stands for our connectedness with Mother Earth.

These four essences form the so-called "circle of fragrances": rosemary (and all the scents related to it) is assigned to the left, bergamot (and all the scents related to it) to the top, geranium (and all the scents related to it) to the right, and patchouli (and all the scents related to it) to the bottom of the quarter circle. In this circle, lavender is assigned to a spot somewhere between bergamot and geranium. We can therefore conclude that lavender, on the one hand, influences our capacity to acknowledge feelings and emotional involvement while it also strengthens our ability to communicate and to respond with greater flexibility.

Martin Henglein has developed and perfected his olfactory tests through trial and error over many hundred experiments. However, it should not be seen as a rigid system, but rather as a flexible frame of reference. In terms of its methodology we could very well compare it to the diagnostic approach in homeopathy. Every essence or blend of essences, containing four oils at the most, finally prescribed, is individually chosen.

About Lavender Martin Henglein says: "Lavender purifies and detoxifies on many different levels. How often was I surprised, even stunned, by the swift healing of wounds that I have observed innumerable times after lavender oil was applied. I use lavender as a prophylactic, for example in cases when there is or has been the danger of an ill-fated crisis in a client's personal development. For me, lavender is the "window to the right decision", because it helps us recognise when we are set in our ways or have got stuck in certain unfounded notions. With the help of its essence we will be in a better position to decide how to get out of any particular cul-de-sac.

"One day one of my clients had to ask himself, if he should master the challenge of the examination to be held the following day. I suggested that before going to bed he should put some drops of lavender oil on a cloth and inhale the vapours. Within minutes his confusion turned to clarity. He was fully aware of his problems and saw clearly that there was only one way to deal with them: he would have to take up the challenge. His worries gone, he had a good night's sleep, and in the morning woke up fully refreshed. It goes without saying that he passed the test".

This small extract from a case history reveals a property of lavender that we can observe time and again: depending on how we feel, its essence can function either as relaxant or as stimulant. Especially in times of internal uncertainty, lavender essence can make us clear thinking and support us to make the right choice.

But Martin Henglein has also used essential oils in his work with mentally retarded patients. His findings are not yet conclusive. In any case, essential oils activate the limbic system, where feelings, long forgotten memories and emotions are stored. Scents thus give us access to this important structure of the brain - and thereby the possibility of helping the mentally retarded in ways that were not open to us before.

No rules are established yet for the vibrational or "subtle body level" of aromatherapy. Guided by their own experiences, aromatherapists follow their intuition, making use of some of the most recent scientific discoveries, while also taking into account their clients' immediate response to the olfactory experience of various essential oils.

In the years to come, the deepening of the already existing communication between aromatherapists around the world will certainly improve research and the practical application of aromatherapy.

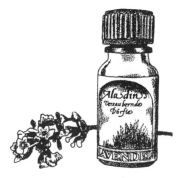

Lavender Recipes

The practical use of lavender oil will enrich your lives, provide for your physical well-being and allow for greater emotional stability. Relaxing baths, massages, compresses, inhalations, aroma lamps in your room, these and other forms of application will all facilitate your enjoyment of the propitious powers inherent in the lavender plant. Although the effects of these powers are undeniable and, if used skilfully, work unfailingly, we still recommend you to seek the advice of an experienced aromatherapist or even a sympathetic medical doctor to discuss your therapy step by step. Should you suffer from serious or chronic symptoms your doctor's advice will be absolutely essential.

After discussing the history and the properties of lavender and its essence, we now want to give you a number of helpful hints as to their actual use in self-healing.

Mind and body are intimately interrelated, so intimately in fact that it would prove difficult to delineate clearly their boundary - to define the dividing line that would separate the one from other once and for all. No matter which you treat first, body or mind, ultimately your treatment will influence both. Of course, not all treatments are equally effective when it comes to modifying or regulating body and mind equally well. Essential oils, however, are. They are a primary example of a genuinely holistic approach. They enter our bodies through skin or nose (for example in a massage or after an inhalation). Via olfactory receptors they finally reach the brain, specifically the limbic system where emotions and memories are stored. From there they influence our state of mind, our mood and disposition. Fragrances can stir up emotions, carry images of the past. They can calm, stimulate, even enchant...

Of the various essences, lavender oil is one of the few which can be applied to the skin in undiluted form, provided no allergic reaction is foreseeable. Essential oils can also be used internally. However, we shall abstain from discussing this form of application, because it should remain solely the responsibility of properly trained and experienced professionals. Besides, even without recipes for internal use we have many suggestions to make, and very often the most gentle and subtle methods are also the most suitable. As repeatedly stated, these methods contribute to the success of aromatherapy in cases of stress. However, we have to participate actively in our own treatment in order to reap the fruit of well-being, equanimity and inner contentment that we strive for. Only active participation in our own aromatherapy will reward us with good and healthy looks and positive personal magnetism.

How to Purchase Lavender Oil

Make sure that you buy pure and 100% natural essences. If that is what the label promises you about a certain oil, take it as a first good sign. However, labels will not always tell the truth. Therefore, do not content yourself with what the label says. Instead, ask your source what kind of lavender was used for distilling this particular oil, where it was grown and how it was processed. Essential oils are similar to wines. There are good years and less good years. So, shop around. Familiarize yourself with different lavender oils, compare them in terms of fragrance and price. The most expensive oil is not automatically the best. But be cautious when you come across "a real bargain", because purity and "bargain prices" may well be mutually exclusive. Remember that over four hundred pounds of lavender are needed to produce just one quart of lavender oil. Wild lavender grown at high altitudes (and especially suitable for use in aromatherapy) takes much longer to harvest by hand than other lavenders that are machine harvested. All these factors contribute to the price. We should take them into account when trying to make up our mind about which kind of lavender oil we should buy. Our final decision, however, should be based on the spontaneous choice of our noses. Label, price and background information are important, but first and foremost we have to like the fragrance of an oil.

The Right Way to Store Lavender Oil

Like any other essential oil lavender oil is best kept in a dark, glass, airtight bottle. If you have purchased a larger quantity, fill what you need of it into a small dropper. The less the oil comes into contact with oxygen the longer it will keep all its properties. Any oxydation adversely affects its quality. Larger quantities of lavender oil should be kept in a cool and dark storage place to further enhance the durability.

Traditionally, in Europe lavender is harvested and distilled between June and August. The new harvest reaches the stores in late September or early October, if not later. This is also the best time to buy a sufficient quantity of your favourite essence and to store it as carefully as you would store a good wine. The optimum time to keep lavender is two years.

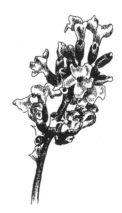

Minor Ailments and Discomforts

Anna Flies to San Francisco

Whilst travelling to San Francisco to give a talk on aromatherapy, across the aisle from me sat a toddler. Anna, a beautiful baby girl, was just over one year old. The ten and a half hours were going to be a long flight for a baby, but for the first few hours Anna remained marvellously composed. How cute she was. Every once and a while I watched her crawling about. But then she got tired and started to cry. A proprietary sleeping draught for babies was administered. This calmed her down, but she still did not sleep, and eventually the calm mood changed to an extremely irritable and noisy one. When picked up she cried, when put down she screamed. If you have ever been on board a plane with a screaming baby, you know how unpleasant this may become: you can't go for a walk to get away from the noise. And we were only half way through the flight! After a while I offered to hold Anna "to give her mother a break", but first I rubbed some lavender oil down my neck. Holding Anna reminded me of my own babies and how lavender had played a big part in their upbringing. Babies grow up, and my family are nearly all teenagers, but lavender remains the same. Within a few minutes Anna was asleep and slept until she was woken up by a stewardess on the approach to San Francisco Airport.

Jet-Lag Bath

Whenever, after a long uncomfortable journey, you feel depressed, bad-tempered and possibly even suffer from an aching back, a stiff neck, and a headache, add these oils to a full bath of water:

lavender	6 drops
marjoram	2 drops
geranium	2 drops

then immediately go to bed.

If you should awaken during the night, put a few drops of lavender oil onto a tissue, settle yourself comfortably and breathe in the vapours, taking slow, relaxed breaths.

Insomnia

Nothing can be more frustrating than going to bed and spending hours thinking about why we cannot fall asleep. In such instances the soothing and pacifying qualities of lavender can bring genuine relief in two seemingly opposite ways: either the effects of the lavender will let us fall asleep gently without even noticing it or they may wake us up so that we can finally think clearly about what is bothering us - putting the matter and ourselves to rest thereafter.

You can achieve this either by impregnating a handkerchief with a few drops of lavender oil and putting it next to you on the pillow so that you can inhale the vapours, or you can use an aroma lamp, or take a bath, adding 5 to 10 drops of lavender oil to a full tub.

Peaceful Sleep, Even for Stressed Executives

One of our friends works for a big company. He travels extensively by car or plane all over Europe, spending every night in a different hotel. One day, he mentioned having difficulties in falling asleep. He said that he just could not detach himself from his work, thinking either about the ramifications of the events of the day that had just passed, or planning for the day to come. We recommended that in the future he should take his aroma lamp with him whenever he travels, to fill it at night with some water and several drops of lavender oil and let the calming, soothing scent fill the air of his hotel room. When we met again, he happily informed us that now he was able to sleep more soundly that he ever had in his whole life.

Muscle Aches and Pains

Every once in a while we get physically exhausted either from sheer exertion or because stress and anxiety are wearing us down. Though after a long hike it may actually be our calves that hurt, the tension caused by psychological uneasiness is usually located in the muscles at the back of our necks, in and around our shoulderblades and trapezius. In this case a relaxing massage may bring relief. However, we do not necessarily have to depend on anybody to give us a massage. We can massage ourselves. Do it, because it will do you a lot of good.

Massage oil for muscle aches and pains

juniper	10 drops
lavender	7 drops
rosemary	8 drops
diluted in 2 fl oz of vegetable oil	

Headaches and Migraine

Lavender can relieve all headaches caused by psychological tension or work-related stress, because it soothes nervous agitation and helps us to relax and let go. A lavender compress applied to the back of the neck or to the forehead will probably lessen or take away the pain within minutes. Just lie down for a moment; apply the compress and breathe slowly and evenly. You may fall aslccp for some minutes. So much the better. Waking up, you will feel refreshed and alive. However, should your headaches be caused by low blood pressure, you would do well to complement the treatment with rosemary baths and a massage with rosemary massage oil. Rosemary is a powerful stimulant for your circulation.

Hypertension

Aromatherapists all over the world prescribe lavender oil against high blood pressure. Lavender baths will also fully support the medical treatment of hypertension. They will help to lower your blood pressure in times of stress and anxiety. In order to bring about the desired effect, you should however make sure that the water temperature is just about or below body temperature.

Bath to Sooth Frayed Nerves

Add to a full tub of water:
lavender	6 drops
marjoram	2 drops
ylang-ylang	2 drops

Chickenpox

A teenage girl contracted chickenpox from a young cousin, whilst visiting relatives. The only essence in the house was lavender. The itching became very intense, but the teenager did not want to scratch for fear of "scarring" herself. The lavender was diluted in water and dabbed onto the spots. This immediately stopped the itching.

Acne

As if to tease us, these annoying little spots and pimples most often mar our faces and torsos in our teenage years when we become aware of our appearance and our looks become a matter of grave importance to us. The changes in our hormonal balance may sometimes even manifest themselves in violent outbursts of acne and a general impurity of the skin.

Fortunately, we can do something about it; for example, counterbalance the hormonal changes by changing our diet, avoiding white flour, sugar and refined foods in general. In addition, we must take good care of our skin. Clogged pores have to be softened up again. Steam baths with camomile or lavender may help, and so will the neat application of lavender oil on afflicted portions of the skin. We just have to put drops of lavender oil on a cotton bud and rub it in carefully. Incidentally, the best time for this is just before going to bed; then, the bactericidal, purifying and regenerating powers of the essence can work overnight. To maximize the benefits, repeat this treatment every other night, until you are satisfied with the results.

Minor Cuts and Scratches

These can be quickly and easily treated with pure lavender essence which is haemostatic, antiseptic and analgesic all in one. Just keep a small phial with lavender oil in your hand-bag in order to be well prepared against minor injuries at all times. Lavender oil should also be a part of your first aid kit when you leave for a long hike into the mountains or anywhere else you may be planning to go.

The Reluctant Cyclist

A friend who, unfortunately, lost his driving licence for a year, and of necessity took to cycling, rather overdid a stint on his bike one day, an exploit which blessed him with a small raw patch of skin on the inside of one buttock. The reluctant cyclist then tried to remedy the problem by sticking a plaster over the sore, in the hope that it would go away. However, as the proverb states: ostriches are in danger even after they have buried their head in the sand. And so was our friend. The annoying sore simply refused to vanish. Worse, it became septic. After one week of suffering he rang to ask me for advice. I suggested gently rubbing one drop of neat lavender oil into the sore with his fingertip. Within days the sepsis had gone and new skin began to grow within the week.

This little story illustrates how the essential oils actually support the powers of self-healing inherent in our bodies: the body is hurt and immediately bacteria from the air take advantage and invade the open wound. The body fights back, causing the typical infection to occur, because the invading bacteria have already overwhelmed the body's front line army. At this point, lavender oil becomes the body's best ally, helping it to push the enemy out. With a little help from the essence, the body itself can "mop up the battlefield and tend to the injured".

The Shaving Accident

Lavender can even help people who do not believe in the power of essences. I have a friend who is a busy city financier and often has to fly overseas for meetings. I had given him a few essences and a brief description of the properties of each, but he remained sceptical.

Early one morning, however, just minutes before the taxi arrived to take him to the airport, he looked in the mirror and saw that he had cut his neck whilst shaving, and his shirt collar was blood stained. He just had time to change shirts; but how was he to stop the bleeding? The essences that I had given him were in the bathroom, and he remembered that lavender oil was the haemostat that he desperately needed right now. He applied a little neat lavender to the wound, and the bleeding stopped immediately - two minutes before the taxi arrived. The next time I saw him, he drily remarked: "Oh, by the way, I had a chance to find out that aromatherapy isn't mumbojumbo."

Insect Bites

Lavender oil can help against the burning and itching of insect bites. I cannot tell you exactly how, but it works. In any event, lavender seems to neutralise the unpleasant stinging that bees, wasps, mosquitos, ants and the like can cause to your skin. If, after an insect bite, your child gets upset and tearful, a drop or two of neat lavender applied directly to the bite and the surrounding area will work wonders. At least that is what I experienced with my own child. No more tears, and no more irritation. However, applied neat, lavender oil does not protect against further bites. If you want to mix your own insect repellant, here is what you do:

Insect repellent	
lavender	10 drops
geranium	10 drops
clove	5 drops
mix with 1 fl oz of jojoba and 1 fl oz of vegetable oil.	

Insects clearly do not like the smell of this, and you will be well protected against future attacks.

Sunburn

Despite all efforts to prevent it, the majority of us have occasionally suffered from sunburn. Feeling sorry doesn't help and neither does chiding ourselves for lack of attention. If sunburn should occur, the first thing to do on returning from the beach is to take a bath to soothe our skin. Fill the tub with water (but make sure that it is not hotter than 70 degrees Fahrenheit) and add 10 drops of lavender and 5 drops of peppermint oil. Since burned skin needs to breathe without impediment, applying fatty oils after the bath will not bring the desired relief. Instead use a cotton cloth and gently dab some diluted lavender oil onto the affected areas. In my experience, the results have always been satisfactory. The sunburn has subsided, and two days later I was out enjoying the sun again and tanning quickly.

Athlete's Foot

If you have been to a public pool or sauna, and two days later feel an itching between your toes, you have probably caught athlete's foot. A number of essential oils will cure it, among them lavender. Just take a cotton bud, put some drops of lavender oil on the tip and dab onto the skin between each toe (two times a day until the fungal infection has improved). Change socks after each treatment.

Skin and Hair Treatment

Facial Scrub

Skin exfoliation is a very popular trend in cosmetics at the moment, and many different commercial brands of facial scrubs are available in stores. However, if you wish, you could easily mix your own individual scrub that would remove dead skin cells just as effectively.

Lavender and oatmeal facial scrub

oatmeal	1 tablespoon
lavender	1 drop

Add sufficient water to make into a creamy (but not too runny) paste. Spread mixture over the face and neck, rubbing gently in circles, paying particular attention to the chin and the area around the nose. Leave for a minute or two, then remove by splashing the skin with cold water. You will find that dead skin cells have been removed whilst the lavender has gently cleansed skin and pores. Your complexion should now be fresh and glowing. Repeat once a week.

Facial Mask

kaolin	1 tablespoon
distilled water	2 tablespoons
clear honey	1/2 teaspoon
lavender	1 drop
geranium	1 drop

Add ingredients to a small bowl and mix thoroughly. The amount should be enough for two applications, and, in the refrigerator, will keep fresh for one week. Honey, geranium and lavender are the ideal ingredients for making your skin smooth and silky.

Eczema

Since birth my little daughter has been suffering from allergy related eczema which was diagnosed early on as some form of constitutional dermatitis. Experience taught me that the scabby rashes appeared most often after consumption of too much sugar and white flour. My daughter is now seven years old and reasonable enough to give up sweets for the sake of the health of her skin. Christmas and Easter, however, are trying times, and the temptations just too numerous. She succumbs and has to pay the price. The itching of her eczema can be very distressing. In one of Maurice Messegué's books on herbal medicine I found the first reference to lavender. Since my daughter's skin was so sensitive, I was not able to use neat lavender oil and decided to make my own cream. In addition, I added lavender oil to her baths. Time and again I saw the she quickly regained the smooth and silky skin of a child.

Lavender Cream

beeswax	2	drams
lanoline (wool fat)	1/2	oz
olive oil	1 1/2	oz
lavender flowers	1	tablespoon
distilled water	1 1/2	fl oz
lavender essence	20	drops

Wax, lanoline and olive oil are melted in a "Bain-Marie". The boiled distilled water is poured over the lavender flowers. Let steep until cool. Strain and add to the fat-oil mixture while stirring continuously with a whisk or electric mixer. As soon as the cream starts to solidify, add the lavender oil. Continue to stir, until the mixture hardens to its final consistency.

Cream in Skin Care

As we all know, cream is the yellowish part of milk, which rises to the top. The word is also used figuratively to describe the best or finest part of something like in "cream of the crop".

When the implications of this simple fact dawned on me, I started to prepare my own creams daily on the basis of cream. This is the most simple recipe you can imagine - fresh and refreshing. Just add one or two drops of lavender oil to one or two teaspoons of cream. Stir briefly and apply to the face.

Treatment for Damaged Hair

Long days in the sun, especially when compounded with repeated baths in the chlorinated water of a swimming pool or in salty sea water at the beach, can put a heavy strain on your hair.

But you can make up to it. Just treat your hair once a week with the following home made oil conditioner.

Treatment for damaged hair

rosewood	15 drops
geranium	5 drops
sandalwood	5 drops
lavender	5 drops
dilute in 2 fl oz of vegetable oil	

Apply carefully with a cotton ball, ensuring that the oil saturates all of the hair, then cover your hair with a towel. After two hours wash and rinse thoroughly.

This treatment is also a good preventative protection and should be applied before you go out to the beach. Apply the oil, and if you like, braid your hair. Your hair will then be well protected against even the most stringent sunbathing and swimming. It will not dry out and it will not bleach.

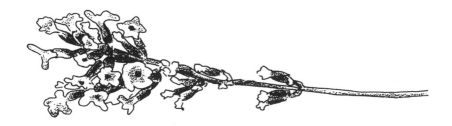

Massage - Touching and Being Touched

Can you imagine anything more beautiful and comforting than being touched? The touch and fragrance of his or her mother -being cuddled, imbibing her reassuring smell - play a primary role in the infant's first perceptions of the world. We remember this throughout our lives and always long to be touched again and to smell the familiar smells we loved. Aromatherapy massage merges these two experiences into a unified experience. An aromatherapy massage rewards both parties involved with the beauty of shared love - rewarding the one who gives as much as the one who receives. And what could be more pleasant or rewarding than the mutual exchange of energy?

Depending on the essential oils we apply, the massage can have very different effects. If we use lavender oil, it will be calming and relaxing, and it will have a soothing effect on the skin. Moreover, lavender oil will encourage the letting go of all muscular tensions, even of the kind that we do not even notice. We can prepare our own pure lavender massage oil or, if we like, add other essences. On page 97 you will find a list of the oils that blend well with lavender. The basic proportion of ingredients is: essential oil 2%, vegetable oil 98% or:

Massage Oil for Relaxation
lavender oil   40 drops
mix with 3 fl oz of vegetable oil

Never pour massage oil directly from the bottle onto the skin, because it will be too cold, and the shock will create additional tension. Instead, put a sufficient quantity into the hollow of your hand, rub your palms to bring to body temperature, and only then touch your partner.

You do not need to have studied massage in order to give a massage. Trust your intuition. Let your hands softly and gently run over the body of your partner. Explore. Find soft and hard spots, and never forget that you want to please, that you want to give something beautiful. Do not try to remember complicated movements like particular styles of kneading and pressing the muscles; if you do it incorrectly, you could harm your partner. Just try to be gentle. This is the best you can do if you are not trained in a certain massage technique. And it works. You will give the gift of comfort and ease - total relaxation.

If you would like to learn massage you might take advantage of any classes available or consult one of the many books, for example Judith Jackson's "Scentual Touch".

Strengthening Your Immune System

A robust immune system can be a great asset when it is damp and cold outside and people are suffering from the flu. It will also help in times of depletion when you are running on empty and are overworked and depressed. An aromatherapy massage will bring much needed relief, and regular massages with fragrant oils will contribute to a strong and healthy immunity. The two oils mentioned in the recipes below are designed for this purpose.

Use them to massage into the back, upper arms, thighs, hands and feet. One session per week will suffice for a general build up of your immune system. However, these massages should be applied daily whenever you are forced to take antibiotics over a long period of time or when you regularly come into contact with somebody who suffers from a cold, a flu or other similar ailment. They will also be of great benefit when you intuitively sense some underlying weakness in you that would make you vulnerable to an infection. In all such cases aromatherapy massage is good preventive care.

Massage Oil I for Strengthening the Immune System

lavender	15 drops
bergamot	5 drops
lemon	5 drops
dilute in 2 fl oz of vegetable oil	

Massage Oil II for Strengthening the Immune System

lavender	10 drops
lemon	5 drops
tea-tree	10 drops
dilute in 2 fl oz of vegetable oil	

By stroking the area around the kidneys you can make them eliminate toxins more efficiently. This massage will also stimulate the function of the adrenal glands, so important for our immune systems. With the flat of both hands massage the kidney area (beginning at the small of the back and spreading to the sides) 15 to 20 times with short, firm, friction strokes. This special kidney massage can easily be integrated into a simple, relaxing massage.

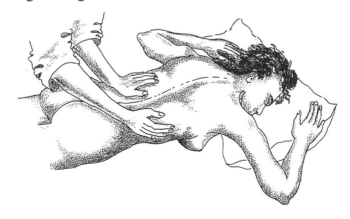

Facial Massage

Facial massages can be tremendously liberating and relaxing. Many memories and emotions are stored in our facial muscles, creating pockets of tension that we never completely release. Together with these muscles, a facial massage may also relax and "thaw" the emotions "frozen" into them. Do not try to hold back any of the feelings that surface. Just surrender to the flow and keep enjoying your massage.

Facial massages are wonderfully relaxing. You can easily get used to them, positively addicted. If you massage your face regularly, it will look more harmonious - "liberated".

Place your hands, palms down, the fingers slightly overlapping in the centre of your forehead. Let the lower hand glide from the eyebrow up to the hairline, while the top hand strokes down from the hairline to the forehead, smoothing it our completely. It is very relaxing and can help prevent headaches.

Massage Oil for the Face (for normal and dry skin)

lavender	10 drops
geranium	2 drops
sandalwood	8 drops
ylang-ylang	5 drops

dilute in 2 fl oz of vegetable, sunflower or almond oil

Especially for Women

Lavender Tampon against Vaginal Discharge

Neat lavender oil on a tampon, inserted at night, will enable you to have a good night's sleep, even if you have a vaginal discharge. This has been known to clear up minor infections within a week. However, if you still have a discharge after this time you should try to find other ways of getting rid of the problem. I would suggest the elimination of coffee and sugary drinks and foods. Stick to bottled water and weak tea. Very often an acute case of vaginal thrush (candida albicans) is brought on by our systems being "overloaded", either by wrong foods, too much alcohol or after taking prescribed drugs. This thrush can then spread to other parts of the body, creating new problems. Because of lavender's anti-inflammatory action, I would recommend the use of lavender oil (20 drops in a cupful of water) to wash the vulva before bedtime and would suggest that advice is sought regarding other essences which may be taken orally.

Mastitis

Mastitis, the inflammation of the mammaries, can be one of the most unpleasant concomitants of breast-feeding. Extreme cases have to be treated with antibiotics which is doubly annoying. In addition to suffering the negative side-effects of the drug, the mother has to stop breast-feeding her baby. Because of the possibly damaging psychological consequences, this can create a most difficult situation. The first symptom usually appears in the form of little red spots. Mastitis may occur when one of the milk ducts get clogged. This can very easily happen if the mother has more milk than the baby needs. Gentle preventive care to clear the milk duct will do what is necessary as long as there is only slight or no fever. Wear your largest bra to give your breasts sufficient space, and ... keep moving. It may sound strange, but cleaning the house, washing dishes, even weight lifting do help, because they actively involve the chest. In addition you can try the following compress:

Compress against mastitis:

rose	2 drops
geranium	1 drop
lavender	1 drop

dilute in 25 fl oz (3 cups) of cold water

Soak the cloth in mixture, wring out and place on chest. Renew application as soon as compress gets warm so that the soothing and antibiotic properties of lavender and rose may take effect.

Post-Natal Depression

The moment a child is born the parents, particularly the mother, have to take responsibility for their baby. Daily chores demand attention and care, and it may take a while and some readjustment to get the situation under control. These sometimes stressful changes, compounded by waking up at night to breast-feed the baby, may actually cause the flow of milk to decline, which in turn may irritate mother and child even more.

In such tense moments it was always a relief for me to put

some drops of lavender oil into the aroma lamp, to inhale the comforting fragrance, and to know that my baby would be comforted too.

Time and again I have heard about lavender healing post-natal depression, soothing frazzled nerves. During the first few days after delivery almost every woman will cry more often than she usually does, because the many new challenges and radical hormonal changes are taxing her energies. She may well be on an emotional roller coaster, euphoric highs changing quickly into a bottomless pit of misery, only to be replaced by yet another unstable high, and the feeling of being out of control may aggravate her even more. In such cases it is best first to stabilise the situation with lavender. After you have regained your composure you can also use some euphorics like jasmine, rose or ylang-ylang either in the aroma lamp, in a bath or by adding some drops to a tissue.

Pets

Elizabeth from the Jersey Lavender Farm told me about the many visitors to the farm, and the many varied ways in which they use lavender. Some people use it to keep fleas out of their homes, others to combat dog fleas. I particularly liked the account of the lady who put some lavender oil around the rim of her bitch's basket during "heat" to disguise that fact from male dogs. Apparently it worked. Even though dogs have a very acute sense of smell the lavender was able to "put them off the scent".

When pets suffer from conjunctivitis, dilute lavender wash may be used on cotton wool to cleanse the eyes. It may also be used for cleaning wounds (after dog or cat fights etc) or for reducing the itching of flea bites.

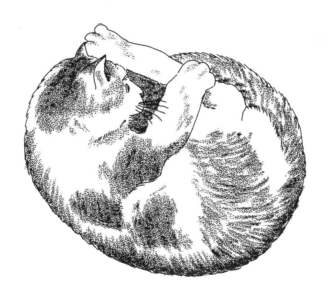

Toilet Training for Kittens

Cats are clean by nature, and kittens are actually toilet trained by their own mothers. However, if you adopt a kitten, it may just forget all its good manners, either because at first it does not find its way around the house or out of protest against the separation from its mother. If your kitten has chosen a spot for relieving itself, it is difficult to change this habit. Smell makes it return to the same place. Essential oils can help to solve the predicament. Just sprinkle the spot with a blend of lavender and peppermint oil. The same blend will also help to prevent your cat sharpening her claws wherever she likes, be it the couch, a cupboard or that beautiful easy chair. Cats have an acute sense of smell and tend to keep clear from all areas scented with strong smelling essences.

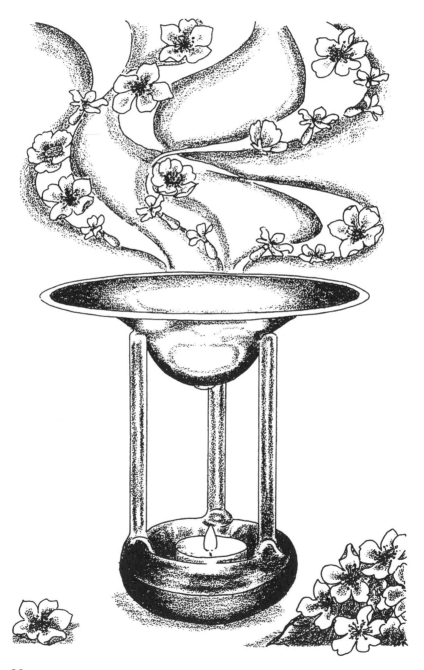

Clearing the Atmosphere

We can use the fragrances which essential oils generate to transform our living or working conditions. Try it. You, your family and your friends will benefit from an environment that brings a sense of relaxation and comfort.

Using the Aroma Lamp

Aroma lamps are a wonderful invention. They make it so easy to subtly perfume a room with just the right dosage of a particular essence or blend of essences. The fragrance will pleasantly permeate the air without assaulting our noses.

There are many different varieties of aroma lamps available commercially; some are electrical while others are powered by candle light. They all function on the same simple principle. A small receptacle which holds the water and the oil is situated above either the light bulb or the candle. The heat of the bulb or candle causes the oil to evaporate, filling the room with its fragrance. The lamps can be a very decorative source of light, made of pottery, porcelain, alabaster or designer glass.

The quantity of oil you use will depend on the size of the room and on the properties of the oil. One or two drops of the heavier essences may well suffice. However, the lighter and more volatile flower - or citrus oil - may actually require as much as 10 to 15 drops. Your nose will indicate the correct amount.

Fragrance influences the atmosphere in a room and the mood of everyone who inhales it. In a public room like an office it would be preferable to use fresh and stimulating oils, whereas in your bedroom you might prefer something with soporific or aphrodisiac qualities.

How We Experience Scents

A better understanding of the physiological processes involved in the perception of these fragrances will give you a clearer idea of their physiological and psychological effects.

Smells influence us, although we may not be aware of it, whether we wish it or not. Since we cannot escape them, we might as well make use of their all-pervasive effects in a positive way. In order to utilise fragrances, we have to know their properties. Does a particular essence release repressed feelings or emotions? Does it enchant us? Will it relax us or liberate us from anxieties or fears?

In some respects our sense of smell is almost primordial. It can transport us instantaneously back into the past. It can fling us far into the future and transform the way we feel here and now. Sounds like magic? It is not. Rather, it is a physiological chain reaction of stunning complexity: through inhalation the odour molecules of the essential oil reach the nasal mucous membrane and its millions of olfactory receptors. With every inhalation approximately 100 million neurons are available to process scent information. These neurons are most intimately and directly connected to the central nervous system. Unlike all other sense perceptions, which are automatically and inevitably filtered through various functions of the brain, scents reach the emotional centre of the limbic system completely uncensored. There they are immediately transformed into relaxing and calming or stimulating and inspiring information, relayed throughout the body and thereby influencing conscious activity and autonomous nervous system alike. In this way, the nose is the only door leading directly to consciousness. Breath is its key.

Lavender - Enchanting and Empowering

Lovely scents entice us to surrender ourselves to the forces of life, filling our breath with vitality. Sounds too mystical and vague? Not necessarily. If we consider how essential oils come into being, their transforming magic will make sense and not appear mystical at all.

Essential oils are "transformed sunlight" or, as one of our friends put it: "fragrant knowledge". This description is actually rather apt. It captures the many different properties of the oils in one encompassing phrase.

As our brief look into the physiological reactions involved in scent perception has revealed, no part of us is left unaffected: fragrances influence us physically and touch us psychologically.

What then is the nature of lavender? How does it influence us? What exactly will its effect on us be? I have tried to describe them in my book *Enchanting Scents*: "Lavender will help us whenever we find ourselves being ruled by Mercury energy instead of commanding it as a servant. In such states, we are generally tortured by fixed ideas; torrents of thought keep us from finding peace, and drive us from one thing to another, like a train speeding across the open landscape. We have hardly taken note of one detail when we are on to the next, and then the one after that. Once Mercury energy is out of control, it seems impossible to bring it to a halt. We have no time to orient ourselves or change our hectic course. The only way to resolve such a situation is to regain tranquillity. In these cases, Mercury energy can only be overcome by Mercury energy. According to Nicholas Culpeper, lavender is ruled by the planet Mercury. In this respect lavender is a wonderful essential oil for inducing the deep, relaxing sleep we need for analysing our situation. Once we have had a good night's sleep in this way, we will be able to differentiate between the positive and negative aspects of Mercury energy in the morning. Our mental clarity will increase and we will find life a lot more enjoyable".

When over-excitement is accompanied by symptoms of mental distress as well as physical pain, lavender oil will transmit the message "relaxation" to all parts of the body. At one time or another the majority of us will have been the victim of blinding headaches caused by nagging thoughts. In these circumstances lavender can bring much needed relief by reprogramming the neurotransmitters involved in the process and thus soothing the overwrought nervous system.

Lavender Does More than Just Relax

In his psychological practice, Martin Henglein rediscovered that lavender can have a rather complex effect on the mental plane, namely that it can be both stimulating and relaxing at the same time. Old herbals confirm this finding. Whenever we have to come to a new understanding of our situation and/or to make an important choice, lavender will help first by stimulating us to solve our problems and get things straight and then by inducing much needed and invigorating rest.

According to Martin Henglein lavender corresponds to "The Lovers" in Tarot, symbolising the reawakening of oneness lost and the abolition of dichotomies - the merging with the flow of actual experience. This picture perfectly captures the effects of lavender on the mental plane.

In *Sounds of Tarot* the German pop group "Merlin's Magic" evokes this plane of experience with their song "Mystery and Key" which is the card of the "Lovers" set to music: "Like a fusion like a dream, making everything so real, she's a mystery to me, she's the key". In the sense of these very words, lavender can be the key to a deeper kind of knowledge. By the way, it can be fascinating to experience music in a room filled with the enchanting scents of essential oils.

Oils Blend with Lavender for the Aroma Lamp

Lavender oil blends well with various other essences. It goes without saying that different combinations will produce different effects. The following recipes are designed for one filling of your aroma lamp. Add the oils from the dropper into the water. If you wish to lay in a small stock of the same blend, just multiply the quantities given here by whatever factor appropriate for your purposes. With some blends, the oils retain their original effects; with other blends a completely new and surprising overall effect is created. We suggest that you first gather some experience with the recipes we give here and then gradually learn to trust your own intuition.

Blend for the Nursery

lavender	5 drops
mandarin	1 drop
rose	1 drop

Blend to induce sleepiness

lavender	10 drops
marjoram	5 drops
niaouli	1 drop

Refreshing Blend

bergamot	5 drops
verbena	5 drops
geranium	3 drops
lavender	2 drops

Relaxing Blend

clary sage	5 drops
lavender	2 drops
ylang-ylang	2 drops
vetiver	1 drop

Blend Promoting Concentration
(ideal for the working space)

verbena	10 drops
grapefruit	2 drops
peppermint	1 drop
geranium	1 drop
lavender	1 drop

Aphrodisiac Blend

ylang-ylang	10 drops
vetiver	1 drop
lavender	1 drop

Asian Blend
for the bedroom

sandalwood	5 drops
jasmine	2 drops
clove	1 drop
lavender	1 drop

Blend for Christmas Season I

mandarin	12 drops
clove	3 drops
lavender	3 drop

Blend for Christmas Season II

mandarin	10 drops
lavender	4 drops
cinammon	4 drops

Blend for Christmas Season III

mandarin	8 drops
lavender	8 drops
jasmin	1 drop

Spring Blend

bergamot	10 drops
neroli	2 drops
ginger	1 drop
lavender	1 drop

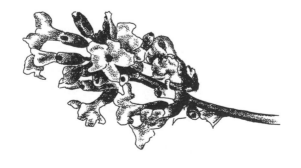

General Effects of Various Essential Oils

(as described in »Enchanting Scents«*)

Bergamot: stimulating; strengthening self-confidence; giving a clearer picture of what the future might hold in store.

Cinnamon: relaxing, can open us to feel sheltered and touched by nurturing warmth.

Clary sage: relaxing, enrapturing, may expand consciousness and give us courage.

Clove: relaxing; may encourage us to let go of behaviour patterns that we have already outgrown, especially in relation to the material plane.

Geranium: stimulating; may harmonize us and at the same time open us to the different rhythms that govern all levels of our lives.

Ginger: stimulates, harmonizes, energizes; may help us to realize aesthetic ideas through creative activity.

Jasmine: strengthens the imagination, putting us into a state of carefreeness, receptivity and buoyancy.

Marjoram: calming; softening sensual input and subduing sexual desire.

Mandarin: overall balancing; improves the ability to approach everyday affairs intelligently.

Niaouli: stimulates sexual awareness, promoting passion, self-abandonment and devotion.

Orange flower: strengthens mental and emotional stability, empowering us with self-confidence and inspiration.

Peppermint:	unclutters the mind, opens new perspectives; strongly enlivening.
Rose:	enticing and stimulating; may make us more active; may strengthen our appreciation of all sensual perceptions while at the same time raising them to the transpersonal level.
Sandalwood:	calming and balancing, sometimes also promoting euphoria; stimulates our imagination and sexual desire, enhances our creativity.
Verbena:	stimulates the mind and our ability to concentrate, accelerates the processing of thoughts, strengthens association and self-confidence.
Vetiver:	balancing; may let us act more assertively, while at the same time raising our level of tolerance and patience.
Ylang-Ylang:	balancing; calms raging emotions, soothes feelings of anger and frustration: liberating and sensually stimulating.

Lavender mixes well with:

bergamot, verbena, geranium, jasmine, camomile, pine, marjoram, mandarin, clary sage, clove, niaouli, neroli, orange flower, rose, sandalwood, grapefruit, peppermint, vetiver, ylang-ylang, cinnamon, stone pine, lemon.

* Monika Jünemann, Enchanting Scents, Lotus Light Publications, Silver Lake, WI, 1989

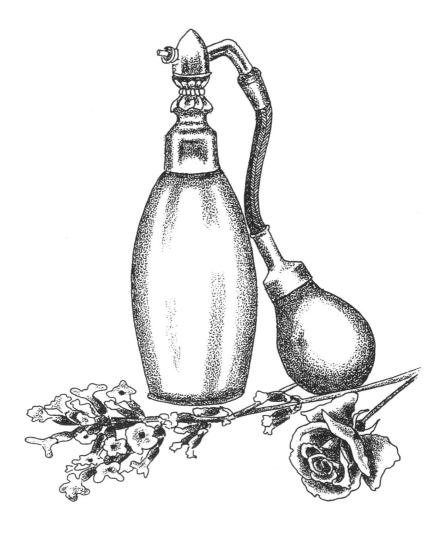

Lavender in Perfumery

Lavender is a favourite material on the perfumer's palette.
The odour of lavender is well known to most of us, whether in our garden or in a luxury soap, Granny's bedroom or in an air freshener. The majority of us can recognize this widely used perfumer's material, but can we describe it? Or more accurately, can we agree on its smell? Lavender has been called: fresh, crisp, sharp, clean, floral, herbal, sweet, green, piney and mossy. Of course, lavender is all of these, but it is also even more. Adjectives alone will not suffice to catch its "essence". It is its diversity or wide "odour profile" that make it such a versatile and popular material for perfumers.

Composing Fragrances

A perfumer is similar to a musical composer. From a simple idea comes a chord followed by a theme. Finally a finished piece is composed using a mixture of logical techniques and inspired, illogical creativity. Good perfumes, whether to adorn a beautiful woman or to accentuate the power of a new bathroom cleaner are, like good music, the result of much work and frustration.

In the creative process the perfumer needs to have certain bench marks that he can relate back to so that he can judge the development of his idea. Lavender is one such bench mark. Others would include rose and jasmine. In other words, these are the major building blocks of perfumery.

The production of lavender as a perfumery material has been dealt with elsewhere in this book. However, it is worth noting that different lavender oils from different geographic locations, and even altitudes, do smell differently, and most perfumers have their individual favourite. In his *Handbook of Perfumery Material* Hugo Janistyn describes some of the peculiarities of different lavender oils:"Essences from the region of Apt markedly smell like mushrooms, an essence from Diois are reminiscent of a particular kind of wild apples, and essences from the region of Luberon are definitely dominated by a green-floral tone..." The English oil, though in short supply, is very different to the continental European product, in that it has a markedly more camphoraceous note. Continental European oils tend to be sweeter and more floral, and are usually offered for sale by their ester content such as 38/40; or 40/42; or 48/50.

From all of this we can conclude that the following simple lavender toilet water would smell quite different if the various qualities of lavender were substituted for one another:

	% by weight
Lavender oil 38/40	70
lavender absolute	10
lemon oil	5
orange oil	5
opoponax extract	2
tonka absolute	3
clove bud oil	1
thyme oil white	1
sage oil	1

In the above formula, lavender is of course the predominant note. The other materials enhance its freshness, sweetness and lasting power in use. Many other materials could be used to enhance various aspects of the odour profile, but few materials could replace lavender.

As well as being indispensible in lavender perfumes, its versatility and wide odour profile make lavender a vital ingredient for virtually all perfume types, from the lightest day perfume to the most seductive and heavy oriental evening fragrance. It can be found in the most exclusive perfumery boutiques and in the humblest of household items in the super-markets.

Lavender as Top and Base Note

Perfumers use lavender as top, middle and base note alike; for the base note the absolute is usually taken. Lavender absolute is obtained not by distillation but by extraction with petroleum ether or other chemical agents. Extracts obtained in this way still contain a lot of flower wax and are called "concretes". After being treated with alcohol, these concretes lose their wax and are called "absolutes".

Sadly, because lavender oil is not the cheapest of materials, it is often substituted in lower-priced perfumes either with its relations, lavandin and spike lavender, or with artificial oils made from synthetic aroma chemicals by perfumers (with the help of chemists). These substitutes are also used in certain applications such as soap, where the delicate nature of real lavender would be ineffective or would be unstable and would produce an "off-odour" during the expected shelf life of the product. So, when a perfumer talks of lavender, he not only means the oil or absolute, but also those materials, natural or artificial, which have a predominantly lavender-like smell.

In alcoholic fantasy perfumery, lavender forms the basis of the "Fougère" type perfume where, with other herbaceous materials and mossy notes, it is widely popular, especially as a masculine perfume. In fact there are few toiletry products tailored to the masculine market which do not contain lavender.

Its fresh herbal aspect allows it to blend with citrus oils such as lemon and lime, other herbs such as rosemary and thyme, and the spice oils like bay and pimento. On the other hand, its sweet woody tones lend themselves to the heavier wood oils such as cedarwood, sandalwood and vetiver. In masculine products a perfumer may use as much as 30% of lavender, but with the exception of lavender perfumes "per se", for feminine fragrances, the percentage of lavender used would be much less, at 5 to 10%. It is for its florality that a perfumer will use it in a feminine perfume to enhance jasmine, rose, lilac and carnation. As in masculine perfumes, it can also be used with the woody oils and with the heavier oriental balsamic notes where it adds to their almost narcotic appeal. This sweetness, particularly of lavender absolute, when used in small traces (less than 1%), is the secret of many successful perfumes.

A Fragrance with Suggestive Powers

In perfumes for cosmetics and toiletries, lavender maintains its importance. "Herbal" or "natural" products often rely heavily on lavender to convey their message, and "medicated" creams and shampoo normally incorporate lavender to reinforce their "do-good" properties. In household products, it is the clean freshness of lavender, acting like the sun on a spring morning, which tells us that the laundry, the bathroom and the kitchen are all as bright as a new pin.

In all the above, lavender is generally used, not in isolation but in combination with countless other materials available to the perfumer. However, it is possible to enjoy lavender on its own. There are several lavender waters and perfumes available. The wide odour profile of lavender allows it to blend with virtually all the other materials available to the perfumer, but supposing one day there were to be no more lavender! Of course, there are the substitutes, but none of them can completely replace the radiance that lavender brings to so many fragrances and products. Without lavender on the perfumer's palette, it would be as though all the greenery of nature were grey and the world a much duller place in which to live.

Composing Your Own Lavender Perfume

"Smells are surer than sounds or sights
to make your heart-strings crack".
Rudyard Kipling

Perfumery has but one goal: to heighten our appreciation of life. - There is no cause nobler than this. The perfumer may spend weeks, months or even years smelling, blending and again smelling various combinations of fragrances. Such a labour of love will eventually produce a new perfume that, novel though it may be, will also seem to be strangely familiar, like an expression in scent of the times in which it was created -like a whiff of a particular "zeitgeist".

How to Blend Your Personal Fragrance

If you simply want to compose your own perfume you do not have to take into account as many factors as does the perfumer. Your task will be easier because you need only please yourself. This is achieved, however, through the same time-honoured methods of traditional perfumery.

The first thing to do is to take some smelling strips. You write the name of the essence to be used on one end and on the other you place a drop of that essence. Then you pick up three strips with different essences and smell them together. If the aroma is not right, you substitute one of the three strips for a different one. This is very easy, fun to do, and an economical way to experiment, because you are not wasting money by adding essences together, which, as a blend, you may not like.

For the final test of a new blend you place two or three drops of it on a cotton tissue and inhale the aroma straight away. Leave for one hour and smell it again. Do you still like the blend?

Lavender Water

Many perfumes and scented waters have disappeared as quickly as they rose to popularity. Not so lavender water and Eau de Cologne which have been popular for centuries. In England for example, lavender water is almost as typically English as high tea and cucumber sandwiches.

Matured after months in alcohol solution, lavender water unfolds its refreshing and stimulating fragrance. Pure lavender waters have something of a classical appeal, an air of conformity, maybe even propriety - worn by women of all ages.

Blended with other oils, lavender quickly loses this air of propriety and reserve. Because of its wide odour profile it does well in almost any combination of oils.

Eau de Cologne

lavender oil	60 drops
bergamot oil	60 drops
lemon oil	50 drops
orange flower oil	50 drops
cinnamon oil	10 drops
rosemary oil	20 drops
in 5 fl oz of 75% alcohol	

Lavender Water

lavender oil	90 drops
lavender absolute	1 drop
rosemary oil	1 drop
orange flower oil	1 drop
geranium oil	1 drop
benzoin absolute (80%)	1 drop
in 3 fl oz of 80% alcohol	

Lavender waters are 90 to 95% alcohol and only 5 to 10% fragrant material and should actually be called "lavender alcohols".

If you feel inspired, you can easily create your own fragrance which will be your own personal statement. Remember the brief descriptions of the oils on page 96. They might well inspire you even further regarding the composition of your blend. And if you find it difficult to procure all the ingredients, don't be shy: get on the phone and call somebody who may be in a position to help. The 'Yellow Pages' with all the business listings in your area are probably all you need to start. Besides, a little research may actually be fun. In the appendix to the book you find additional adresses and sources of supply.

Lavender Perfume

To obtain a lavender perfume you increase the proportion of fragrant materials to 15 to 30% of the total volume of your blend (i.e 25 to 50 drops of essential oil in 1/2 fl oz of carrier fluid). Ideal carrier fluids are high grade ethyl alcohols, or preferably liquid waxes like jojoba oil which will be kinder to your skin than alcohol.

Start with simple combinations consisting of three oils: one base, one middle and one top note. They will be the founding chord of your composition.

Top notes are light and most volatile. Middle notes are warm and mild. Base notes are heavy, deep and sustained vibrations. Together they make a perfect "chord".

The essence of lavender can potentially be used in all three notes. If it contains more than 50% ester, it can be a top note. If it contains less than 50% ester, it can be a middle note, and as absolute, it is a suitable base note. To compose your own lavender perfume you may choose from among these top, middle and base notes:

Top Notes	Middle Notes	Base Notes
lavender oil	lavendin oil	lavender absolute
bergamot oil	lavender oil	rosewood oil
verbena oil	rose oil	patchouli oil
lemongrass oil	geranium oil	benzoin absolute
lemon oil	jasmine absolute	sandalwood oil
peppermint oil	neroli oil	vetiver oil
mandarin oil	clary sage oil	oak moss absolute
	birch oil	tonka absolute
	rosemary oil	honey absolute

Of top and middle notes you take more, of base notes less.

Let us assume that you would like to obtain a perfume of the "Fougère" type. For this you would need a fresh, herbal lavender and a mossy background, paraphrased with one or two drops of another top, middle or base note. The following "Fougère" would be a good model on which to base your endeavours.

Fougère Privée (feminine)

lavender oil 48/50	20 drops
lavender oil 30/32	10 drops
lavender absolute	1 drop
honey absolute	1 drop
neroli oil	1 drop

in 1/2 fl oz of 90% ethyl alcohol or 1/2 fl oz of jojoba oil

Many variations are possible. You can add sweet oils to accentuate the feminine character; you can add some oriental perfume to make the blend appear heavier and aphrodisiac, or you can add more austere woody notes for a men's perfume.

"Fougère"-Privée (oriental)

lavender oil 48/50	20 drops
bergamot oil	15 drops
neroli oil	5 drops
patchouli oil	1 drop
jasmine absolute	2 drops
honey absolute	2 drops
tonka absolute	1 drop

in 1/2 fl oz of 90% ethyl alcohol or 1/2 fl oz of jojoba oil

"Fougère"-Privée (masculine)

lavender oil 48/50	30 drops
birch oil	10 drops
verbena oil	2 drops
oak moss absolute	2 drops
benzoin absolute	1 drop

in 1/2 fl oz of 90% ethyl alcohol or 1/2 fl oz of jojoba oil

And Finally Some Psychology

Whenever we try to define the fragrance of the different kinds of lavender conclusively, we run into the problem of the plant's obstinate resistance to all such attempts.

In the chapter on aromatherapy we already stated that lavender essence can have both calming and stimulating effects. In his research on the psychology of scent, the perfumer Paul Jellinek tried to find some more precise answers. He differentiates between lavender essences, obtained from the whole plant through steam distillation, and the so-called lavender flower oils, which are actually extracts and known as absolutes. According to his findings both materials have calming and soothing effects. The essential oil has a basically refreshing effect; although, because of its linalool, it is also slightly narcotic. The absolute is more markedly narcotizing and has a more flowery smell. However, the large group of terpene alcohols also contained in lavender oil cannot be properly categorized because of their wide range of effects. They can be either anti-erogenous, narcotic or erogenous.

Since so many different factors are involved, the psychological effects of lavender are hard to generalize. Being unique itself, each essence will naturally also be unique in its effects; and, depending on what kind we choose, it may either stimulate our sexual appetites or dampen them.

Most of us are not chemists and do not have the equipment needed for a reliable chemical analysis of lavender oils. We have to trust our noses and let experience be our teacher. Even so, venturing into the domain of the perfumer can be a lot of fun.

How to Cultivate Your Own Lavender

If you decide to grow your own lavender plants, the first decision is whether to grow from seed or from a nursery cutting. There are numerous places where lavender plants may be purchased, and the advice of a grower should be sought as to the type of lavender you are acquiring. A plant which is fragrant and has purple flowers should ensure a good essential oil content. Growing from seed will naturally take longer, but it does make it possible to choose the exact cultivar that you want by name. For instance, in the "Suffolk Herbs Catalogue", there is a choice of six different lavenders, and if I wished to cultivate lavender from seed I would choose *lavendula vera*.

After you have made your choice, the next step is to prepare the soil. Lavender is a hardy plant, and once the basic requirements are attended to, it needs very little attention during the year. It likes a light, well-drained, alkaline soil and should be planted in a sunny position. If the soil is too rich or heavy, it can be made lighter by the addition of sand. Remember that lavender grows wild on mountain sides where rainwater naturally drains away. It will not grow on clay based soils, but a chalky soil such as that on the southern English coast is ideal.

Fertilizer is not necessary for the first few years, but when used it should be applied in November rather than in spring.

Potash is recommended as it encourages flower development. As lavender can easily become overwhelmed by weeds, occasional hoeing will ensure that the lavender plants are not being robbed of vital nutrients. The failure of a single lavender plant, or even of an entire plantation, could be due to a poorly drained soil, as pools of stagnant water remaining on the ground are injurious to lavender.

Weather

If you are planning a herb garden, please do give lavender the sunniest spot, as the more sun it receives during the summer months, the more aromatic your harvest will be. Many other herbs require direct sunshine, but it should be possible to combine them to advantage. The Elizabethans planted "knot gardens" where the lavender formed a wall, surrounding a selection of other aromatic plants.

In its natural habitat of Southern France lavender is known to be hardy. It can withstand both the low temperatures of winter and the hot summers. And yet it can suffer from weather-related problems. A dry spring may hinder the development of young shoots. This problem can be overcome, however, by simply watering the plants in your herb garden, an impracticality on a larger lavender plantation. There is another weather problem which cannot be guarded against, however. A severe spring frost could kill your plants.

Heavy and prolonged rainfall any time in June when the spikes first appear, until the crop is harvested in July and August, can result in the loss of as much as 90% of the oil yield. Conversely, according to Norfolk Lavender, an exceptionally fine summer like that experienced in England during 1989 can have the effect of increasing the yield by as much as 50%.

Propagation

Lavender can be propagated either sexually (by seeds) or asexually (by cuttings). Seeds from hybrids will produce mixed flowers but growing from seeds is much cheaper and possibly more rewarding emotionally. The seeds need to be kept warm and moist. As they have a very hard covering, several months may pass before they germinate. The time for planting lavender seeds is either March or April.

Propagation by cuttings is known as "clonal" propagation and ensures that plants are of uniform size and height. This is of paramount importance to commercial lavender growers and would be important for you, if you were growing a lavender hedge or "knot garden". Cuttings are taken in April or October by pulling off side shoots about 6 inches long, downwards, so that they tear away some of the old wood where it joins the main branch.

These should be planted so that 3 inches of new growth remains visible, and then tread down. It is important to plant cuttings in a nursery bed so that they can be covered with polythene during the cold winter. At Norfolk Lavender, cuttings will always spend their first winter under polythene to give them a measure of protection from frost and snow.

Thousands of hybrids can be obtained by growing from seed, and many people have lavender plants named after them. Clones that become horticulturally important are known as cultivars and named according to the *International Code of Nomenclature Cultivated Plants*.

Disease

The most virulent killer of lavender is *Phoma Lavendulae* (also known as "shab"), which is a parasite fungus. First definite signs of infection appear in late spring, when the young shoots turn yellow and die in isolated patches. Once the fungus is visible, it will spread downwards and kill the plant, after which it will probably spread to other nearby lavenders. There is no known cure. Some cultivars are more resistant than others. According to Henry Head of Norfolk Lavender (who has watched a 50 acre field die within a two year period), the closer the lavender hybrid is genetically to *Lavendula angustifolia*, the more resistant it is to disease; the closer the hybrid is genetically to *Lavendula latifolia*, the more susceptible to disease it appears to be.

If we look at the chapter dealing with the chemistry of lavender, we will see that the chemical constituents of spike lavender are different to those of "true" lavender. We might therefore suppose that "true" lavender contains a chemical or a group of chemicals which protects the plant from fungus and that, as the lavender is hybridized with spike, this protection is bred out of the plant. Should your plants develop shab, try spraying them with a dilution of tea tree oil in water. I cannot give any guarantees, but tea tree is a known anti-fungal agent, and has helped human fungal infections such as *Candida albicans*. So it may just work on plants as well.

Insects (pests) can also be a problem, but at least these can be removed from individual shoots before they cause too much harm. In Tasmania the principle pest is a small moth whose larvae attack the lavenders when the springtime shoots appear. Left unchecked, the moths will defoliate the plants and kill them. Another pest is the caterpillar of a tiny butterfly which eats the flowers. Occasional inspection of the plants in the spring will show whether there is any unwelcome insect which needs to be removed immediately.

Pruning

Lavender thrives on hard cutting and should be cut back as soon as the crop is taken. If plants are allowed to develop freely they will become leggy and debilitated in about seven years. Annual pruning will help the plant to retain its vigour and shape.

Harvest

Some lavender growers say that the plants should be harvested just before the flowers are open; but as the linalyl acetate is at its maximum when the flowers are in bloom, the essential oil will not have developed to its optimum. If on the other hand the flowers are left on the plants too long, they begin to dry out and will then drop off onto the ground. A friendly visit to your plants each day during July will soon let you know when the time is right. Your nose will tell you.

Drying

Essential oil loss could be as high as 24% after drying the lavender in full sunlight and between 2-10% when drying lavender in the shade.

To dry lavender tie it into bunches and suspend it from the ceiling. Be sure to place a sheet of paper underneath to catch any falling flowers. The harvested plants can also be spread onto a sack or wooden shelf, in which case, they will have to be turned over everyday. The room needs to be dry and airy, and the drying completed as soon as possible. Careful handling is important because, if the flower heads are rubbed, the oil glands will break and the essential oil will be released. Carefully dried lavender flowers, for use in potpourris or sachets, will retain their colour and fragrance for several years.

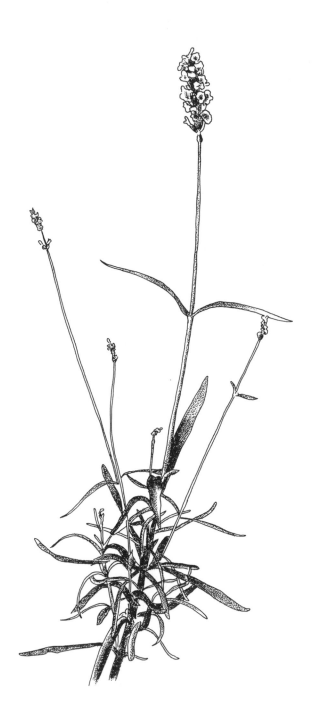

114

Odds and Ends...

Many varied and beautiful things can be made with lavender. If you love flowers and fragrances, you will also love lavender; you can use its purple spikes to decorate your house or apartment or add its flowers to a potpourri.

A lot can be learned about the art of arranging and combining different fragrant flowers from ancient herbals, and it is great fun to dip into these heavy old texts or their modern reprints.

Memories are imbued with smells, so much so that smells inevitably evoke memories. Potpourri is a wonderful way of bringing back the memory of spring and summer to duller autumn and winter days.

Potpourri

Provided your recipe is correct, preparing your own potpourri is actually quite easy. You need good ingredients: dried flowers, herbs, some kind of fixative, essential oils, and possibly a few additional components. These are mixed together and placed in a decorative container.

For centuries lavender flowers and lavender oil have been among the most popular potpourri ingredients. However, if you want to enjoy your potpourri for months and even years to come, you must master the art of its composition. But first it is essential to ensure the quality of the ingredients you use.

There are wet and dry potpourris. Wet potpourris are traditionally the oldest but are also more difficult to make. So, if you do not have any experience in making potpourris, you should start with a dry potpourri.

The process is always the same. Mix the dry components which must be absolutely dehydrated, taking care not to break the sensitive flower skins, and add the essential oil. To give it time to mature, the mixture is stored for two weeks in an airtight container, preferably in a dark cool place. From time to time the ingredients may be stirred cautiously to ensure a harmonious blending of all fragrances. After two weeks the potpourri is ready to be put into a bowl or basket and placed in a desirable position.

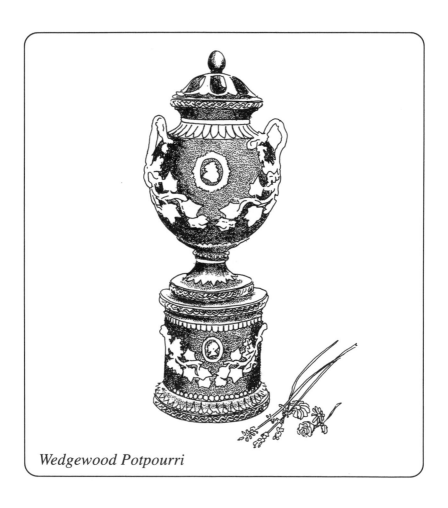

Wedgewood Potpourri

Lavender Potpourri

lavender flowers	7 oz
wild mallow flowers	3 oz
cornflowers	1 oz
whole cloves	1 oz
quills of cinnamon	1 oz
ground cloves	1/2 oz
ground cinnamon	1/2 oz
ground orris root	1 oz
lavender oil	25 drops

This is a variation of a traditional potpourri. Violet lavender, dark purple mallow, and blue cornflowers merge to provide a beautiful "serenade in blue". Of course, you can use the same proportion for other ingredients as well. A good fixative is absolutely essential for durability. If desired, you can replace orris root with benzoin resin, vertiver or storax, the ground root of Florentine sword flag or oak moss.

If your potpourri begins to lose its fragrance just add some drops of essential oil.

Potpourri Grasse

lavender flowers	7 oz
patchouli leaves	3 oz
hibiscus flowers	2 oz
rose flowers	2 oz
anise	1 oz
ground rosemary	1/2 oz
cedarwood	2 oz
ground orris root	1 oz
lavender oil	20 drops
patchouli oil	10 drops

This potpourri may bring back the smells of Grasse as they filled the streets of this ancient town in southern Provence when ships from the Orient brought spices and fragrant oils for local perfumeries. Its calming oriental-provencal fragrance still has the power to sooth us in the more hectic days of the modern era.

Pomander

I saw my first pomander near Findhorn Bay in Scotland. I had entered a house in a village to ask for directions and wondered why this woman was loading the orange she had in her lap with cloves. When I asked her, she told me about pomanders, adding that she liked to suspend them from her kitchen walls during the cold days in winter. They would fill the air with their pleasant perfume even with the window closed. The aroma in her room was convincing evidence of this.

In the so-called good old days, pomanders were precious balls made of ivory, gold or silver, richly decorated with filigree patterns and filled with spices and animal fragrances as fixatives. Today, we use oranges, lemons, limes instead, load them with scented cloves and then dry them by placing them in a mixture consisting of various spices. The fruits shrivel and harden. This process always reminds me of the mummifying of corpses in ancient Egypt which was achieved by completely dehydrating the dead body with natron and the help of various essential oils. Bactericidal and fungicidal substances in the essential oils then prevented any further decomposition caused by bacteria. In pomanders, the essential oils fundamentally work in the same way; the other spices only enhance the fragrance.

Lavender Pomander

orange	1
cloves	100-200
lavender oil	30 drops

Place cloves in airtight container, add lavender oil and close the lid. Let the cloves quietly absorb the oil for one or two days, then load the orange. The cloves should be placed close together but not touching one another. You can cover the whole orange with these cloves. However, should you wish to hang it up, you need to leave two strips free for the ribbons. After covering the pomander with the cloves place it in the following spice mixture:

ground cinnamon	2 oz
ground cloves	1 oz
ground nutmeg	1/6 oz
ground orris root	1/2 oz

Mix the spices and pour some of the mixture into the dish, place the pomander on top and cover with the remainder of the spice mixture. Depending on its size, preservation will take from two weeks to a month. While it is drying the pomander should be turned occasionally. Afterwards the fruit will be much smaller and very hard.

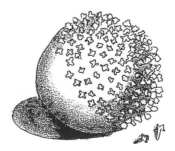

Lavender Sachets

Sachets are placed in cupboards and drawers to impregnate linen, towels, quilts, lingerie, outerwear, or whatever you wish, with their fragrance. Their size is such that they can easily be slipped into your wardrobe or chest of drawers.

Lavender sachet		
starch	3	oz
ground orris root	1/2	oz
lavender oil	15	drops

Pour starch or talcum powder into a flat dish, add lavender oil, and blend well with your fingertips. Then fill sachet. If you do not have one readily available, you can easily make one. Take a piece of densely woven cloth 20" x 2", fold and sew lengthwise, turn outside in so that the seam disappears, and fill sachet with the help of a funnel. Finally you can tie the sachet with a pretty ribbon.

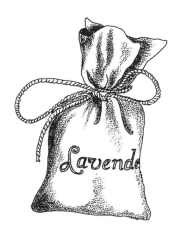

Moth Sachets

In a variation of the above recipe you can make your own moth-repellent sachets. Instead of 15 drops of lavender oil you add 10 drops of pine tree oil and 10 drops of lavender oil to the powder. In the old days linen chests were often made from pine wood, and the moth problem was solved automatically.

Lavender Pillow

A lovely way to enhance your sleep is to scent your pillow with lavender. There are many possible ways to do this.

Place a cotton ball scented with lavender oil among your pillows.

Take two rectangles of wool or loden material. With right sides together, sew around three of the edges. Turn the bag the right way out and fill with lavender flowers and cotton balls soaked with lavender oil. This small pillow can be sewn into a cover of some finer material, like muslin, silk or lightweight cotton. When the fragrance becomes weaker, just squeeze hard or add more scented cotton balls.

Sew pillows of different sizes which you can embroider or mark with dye and fill with lavender flowers. If you put the flowers into a woollen inlay, your pillow will not make any rustling noises which would prevent you from sleeping. Made in attractive fabrics, these pillows make ideal presents.

Scented cushions which match the design or fabric of an easy chair are called "saddle-bags". Like a saddle bag on a horse, they are hung over the back of a chair. They are filled with different blends of fragrant material so that anyone sitting in the chair will be surrounded by a pleasantly fragrant aura.

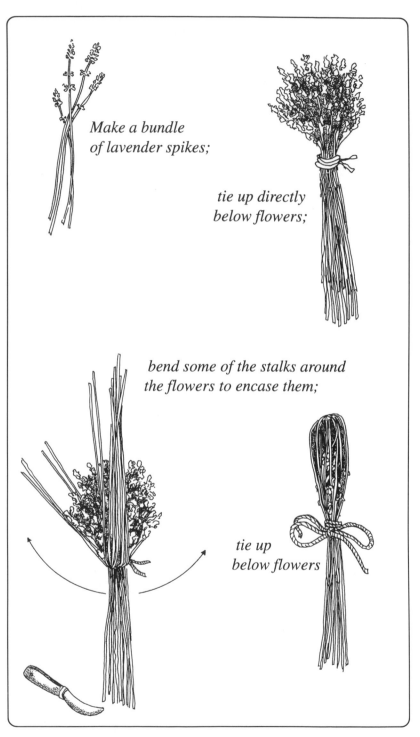

Make a bundle
of lavender spikes;

tie up directly
below flowers;

bend some of the stalks around
the flowers to encase them;

tie up
below flowers

"Faggots"

When you have grown your own lavender, cut off several stems and remove the leaves while the plant is in bloom. Then tie a thread around the bunch, just below the flowers, and bend the stems around the flowers so that the flowers are encased in stems. The stems are then secured with thread and the "faggot", as it is called, is left to dry. Once dry, interlace the stems with a length of very thin lavender coloured ribbon. In France and England, the two traditional "lavender countries", these "faggots" used to be very popular. Now they are also made in Japan, where potpourries and herbs are experiencing much popularity.

... And the Like

In Winter you can drop two drops of lavender onto some pine cones and then burn them in an open fireplace or wood-burning stove. The delightful fragrance will fill the room. As a further experiment, add lavender and cinnamon, or lavender and orange, or lavender and clove to your pine cones.

Since lavender oil does not leave any grease spots, you can put some drops on the paper on the bottom of your linen drawers. Or you can use lavender together with other kinds of oil for freshness and fragrance.

The suction fan feeding the air fan of ionizers is usually covered with some kind of foam. Just put some drops of lavender oil on it, and the aroma will subtly fill the room.

In some flea markets you can still find scent dispensers made from unglazed pottery. If you fill them with lavender oil, the fragrance will evaporate through the porous sides of the dispenser.

Even the stalks of the lavender plant contain some essential oils. Do not throw them away after you have used the flowers for potpourris and the like. Instead tie them together with a nice ribbon and place them wherever seems fit: in shoe boxes, in the attic of your house. Broken down to size, they can also be added to sachets.

You can also prepare your own furniture polish. Add 1/6 oz of beeswax to 2 oz of soya oil. Melt wax and oil in a "Bain-Marie" and add 10 drops of lavender oil. Stir until cold and hardened and put into a container with a tight lid. This polish should be used sparingly. After application, polish furniture with a woollen cloth.

To make your own lavender starch: pour 3 oz of rice starch, .5 teaspoon of borax, 1/2 teaspoon stearic acid into a mortar, add 10 drops of lavender oil and blend thoroughly with a pestle. Use 3 teaspoons per washing machine and 1 tsp per hand basin.

If you dry your laundry in a dryer, you can add a cloth impregnated with essential oils: lavender for kitchen cloths and towels; for bedspreads and covers use lavender, rose, jasmine or ylang-ylang; for men's wear use cedarwood or vetiver. Make sure that for each oil you use a different cloth so that each piece of laundry is scented appropriately.

Scented ink is a romantic way of writing a letter to a loved one. Add a few drops of lavender essence to a small pot of ink (any colour you like, but preferably a light blue) until the scent is just right. Then add water to make the colour more subtle.

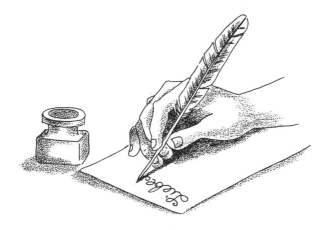

Table of Suggested Applications of Lavender Oil

	apply neat:	aroma lamp:	compress:	dilute wash:	douche:	eye bath:	facial massage:	herb pillow:	inhalation:	massage:	mouthwash:	on cotton wool:	on tampon:	perfume:	sitzbath:
acne					●		●								
air purifier		●													
anxiety		●						●						●	
athlete´s foot	●														
bad breathe				●											
burns (first aid)			●												●
chickenpox				●											
colds									●						
conjunctivitis						●									
convulsions			●												
croup									●	●					
cuts (first aid)	●			●											
cystitis				●											
ear ache												●			
eczema				●											
fever			●	●											
gum (bleeding/soreness)	●			●								●			
headache		●	●												
heat rash				●											
hypertension		●						●							
immunity (low)										●					
influenza		●													
insect bites	●														
insomnia	●		●												
jet lag															
leucorrhea					●										

Table of Suggested Applications of Lavender Oil

	apply neat:	aroma lamp:	compress:	dilute wash:	douche:	eye bath:	facial massage:	herb pillow:	inhalation:	massage:	mouthwash:	on cotton wool:	on tampon:	perfume:	sitzbath
muscular aches										●					●
muscular cramps										●					●
mouth ulcers	●										●				
nosebleeds	●														
period pains			●												
pet care				●											
pierced-ear soreness	●														
scar tissue										●					
skincare							●								
snake bites (first aid)	●														
spots and pimples	●						●								
sterilising tweezers etc.	●														
stress		●							●	●					●
stretch marks										●					
teething babies															●
thrush (vaginal)					●								●		
toothache			●												
travel sickness									●						
wound cleansing				●											

Compress:	Add 3-4 drops of lavender oil to a bowl of hot water. Dip clean cloth in liquid, squeeze excess, apply.
Douche:	Add 20 drops of lavender oil to warm water, mix well.
Eye bath:	Add 1 drop of lavender oil to 1 cup of tepid water, mix well, pour sufficient quantity into eye bath.
Herb pillow:	Put a small pillow of lavender flowers under your normal pillow or add a few drops of lavender oil to the edge of your pillow.
Inhalation:	3-4 drops in bowl of hot water. Cover head and bowl with towel and breathe deeply for five minutes.
Internal:	1 or 2 drops on small spoonful of sugar, or in small glass of honey water.
Massage:	2% lavender oil (or combination of lavender and other essences) in vegetable oil.
Perfume:	Mix 5 drops of lavender oil into 100 drops (1 teaspoonful) of jojoba oil and apply to wrists and neck.
Sitz bath/bath:	Add 6 drops of lavender essence to bidet or bowl of water (sitz bath), for a bath: 6 dops to full tub – mix well.
Tampon:	Put a few drops of lavender on tampon, insert at night-time.

Lavender Farms to Visit

(July and August only)

Norfolk Lavender
Caley Mill
Heacham
Kings Lynn
Norfolk, England

The Jersey Lavender Farm
Rue de Pont Marrquet
St Brelades
Jersey

Bibliography

English Language Works

Amerding, George: *The Fragrance of the Lord*, San Francisco, 1979

Beedell, Suzanne: *Herbs for Health and Beauty*, Sphere Ltd., 1972

Bethal, May: *The Healing Power of Herbs*, Wilshire Book Co., Wilshire, Calif., 1973

Bremness, Leslie: *The Complete Book of Herbs*, Dorling, Kindersley, 1988

British Herbal Pharmacopeia, British Herbal Medicine Association, 1979

Clark, Oliver: *Never Catch Colds Again*, Health Science Press, 1979

Colin, Claire: *Of Herbs and Spices*, Abelard Schumann, 1961

Culpeper, Nicholas: *Culpeper's Complete Herbal*, W. Foulsham & Co.

Duke, James: *A Handbook of Medicinal Herbs*, CRC Press, 1929

Gattefossé, René-Maurice: *Formulary of Perfumery and Cosmetics*, Chemical Publishing Company, New York, 1959

Genders, Roy: *History and Scent*, London 1972

Griggs, Barbara: *Green Pharmacy*, Jill Norman & Hobhouse, 1981

Guenther, Ernest: *The Essential Oils*, D. van Nostrand & Co. Ltd., 1952

Hemphill, Rosemary: *The Penguin Book of Herbs and Spices*, 1966

Heriteau, Jacqueline: *Potpourris and other Fragrant Delights*, Penguin, 1978

Hills, Lawrence: *Herb Growing the Organic Way*, Henry Doubleday Research Association, 1983

Humphrey, John: *The Pharmaceutical Journal of Formulary*, The Pharmaceutical Journal Office, 1904

International Journal of Aromatherapy, Vol. 1, No. 2. The Tisserand Aromatherapy Institute

Kirihara, Haruko, *Herbal Craft*, 1988

Law, Donald: *Herbal Teas for Health and Pleasure*, Health Science Press, 1968

Lawrence, Brian/Tucker, Arthur: "Herbs, Spices, and Medicinal Plants - Recent Advances in Botany", *Horticulture and Pharmacology*, Vol. 2

Leung, Albert: *Encyclopedia of Common Natural Ingredients Used in Food, Drugs and Cosmetica*, John Wiley & Sons, 1980

Levy, Juliette de Bairacli: *The Illustrated Herbal Handbook*, Faber & Faber, London, 1974

Lucas/Stevens: *Book of Recipes*, J & A Churchill

Mills, Simon: *The Dictionary of Modern Herbalism*, Thorsons, 1985

Maury, Marguerite: *Guide to Aromatherapy*, C.W Daniels, Saffron Walden, 1989

Potters New Encyclopedia, Health Science Press, 1907

Presting, Sally:*The Story of Lavender*, Heritage in Sutton Leisure

Ramstad, Egil: *Modern Pharmacognosy*, McGraw-Hill, New York, 1959

Rimmell, Eugene: *The Book of Perfumes*, Chapman & Hall, 1865

Rose, Jeanne: *Your Natural Beauty*, Kerats Publ., 1978

Rovesti, Paolo: *Of Perfumes Lost*

Sagarin, Edward: *The Science and Art of Perfumery*

Stanway, Andrew: *Alternative Medicine*, Penguin, 1980

Thomsons, C.J.S: *Mystery and Lure of Perfume*, Bodley Head, 1929

Tisserand, Robert: *Aromatherapy: To Heal & Tend the Body,* Lotus Press, 1988

Toller, S/Dodd, G: *Perfumery - The Psychology and Biology of Fragrance*, Chapman & Hall, 1988

Trease, G.E/Evans W.C: *Pharmacognosy*, 1934

Wagner H/Bladt S/Zagindski E.M: *Plant Drug Analysis*, Springer, 1983

Walker, Benjamin: *Encyclopedia of Metaphysical Medicine*, Routledge & Kegan Paul, 1978

White, Edmund/Humphrey, John: *Pharmacopeia*, 1901

Wise, Rose: "Flower Power", Nursing Times, May 1989

French Language Works

Balz, Rudolphe: *Les Huiles Essentielles*, 1986

Meunier, Christiane: *Lavandes et Lavendins*, Edisud, Aix-en-Provence, 1985

Rouviere, Andre/Meyer, Marie-Claire: *Les Huiles Essentielles*, M.A Editions, 1983

Thau, Jeannine Pierre du: *D'Autres Souvenirs de la Cité des Parfumes*, Nizza, 1986

German Language Works

Breindl, Ellen: *Das große Gesundheitsbuch der Hildegard von Bingen*, Paul Pattloch, Aschaffenburg, 1983

Freud, Sigmund: *Gesammelte Werke in chronologischer Ordnung*, Band 7, London, 1941

Gildemeister, Eduard: *Die ätherischen Öle*, Akademie Verlag, Berlin 1956

Horn, Effi: *Parfüm - Zauber und Geheimnisse der Duftstoffe*, Verlag Mensch und Arbeit, Munchen, 1967

Janistyn, Hugo: *Handbuch der Kosmetika und Riechstoffe in 3 Bänden*, Heidelberg, 1969-1978

Jellinek, Paul: *Praktikum des modernen Parfümeurs*, Alfred Huthig Verlag, Freiberg, 1960

Jellinek, Paul: *Parfüm und Eros*, Baierbrunn, 1980

Jellinek, Paul: *Die psychologischen Grundlagen der Parfümerie*, Alfred, Huthig Verlag, Heidelberg, 1965

Jung, Carl Gustav: *Mysterium Coniunctionis*, Gesammelte Werke Band 14/2, Walter Verlag, Olten

Jubeczka, K.-H.: *Vorkommen und Analytik ätherischer Öle*, Thieme Verlag, Stuttgart, 1979

Launert, Edmund: *Parfüm und Flakons*, Callway, München, 1985

Launert, Edmund: *Duftspendende Pflanzen*, Baierbrunn, 1985

Müller, Irmgard: *Die pflanzlichen Heilmittel bei Hildegard von Bingen*, Otto Müller Verlag, Salzburg, 1982

Müller, Arno: *Die physiologischen und pharmakologischen Wirkungen ätherischer Öle*, Heidelberg 1951

Reger, Karl-Heinz: *Hildegard-Medizin*, Goldmann Verlag, München, 1984

Treffer, Gerd:*Grasse - Stadt in der Provence*, Bamberg, 1980

Suggested Reading

Jackson, Judith: *Scentual Touch - The Time Honoured Art of Massage with Fragrant Oils and Herbs*, Fawcett Columbine, New York, 1986

Jünemann, Monika: *Enchanting Scents - The Secrets of Aromatherapy*, Lotus Light, Wilmot, WI., 1988

Maury, Marguerite: *Guide to Aromatherapy - The Secret of Life and Youth*, C.W Daniel, Saffron Walden, 1989

Price, Shirley: *Practical Aromatherapy - How to Use Essential Oils to Restore Vitality*, Thorsons, Wellingborough, 1987

Tisserand, Maggie: *Aromatherapy for Women*, Thorsons, Wellingborough, 1985 and 1990

Tisserand, Robert: *The Art of Aromatherapy*, C.W Daniels, London 1977

Tisserand, Robert: *Aromatherapy: To Heal & Tend the Body,* Lotus Press, Twin Lakes, WI, 1988

van Toller, Steve & Dodd, George (eds.): *Perfumery - The Psychology and Biology of Fragrance*, Chapman & Hall, London, 1988

Valnet, Jean: *The Practice of Aromatherapy*, C.W Daniels, Saffron Walden, 1980

Addresses and Sources of Supply

Wholesale
(Contact with your business name, resale number or practioner license)

LOTUS LIGHT
PO BOX 1008 ML
Silver Lake, WI 53170
414/889-8501
Fax 414/889-8591

Retail
Lotus Fulfillment Service
33719 116th Street Box ML
Twin Lakes WI 53181

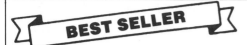
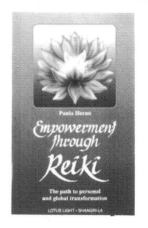
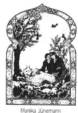
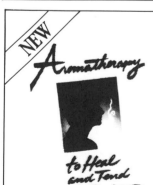

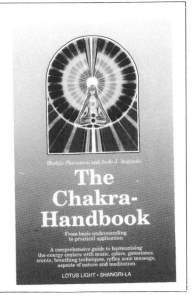
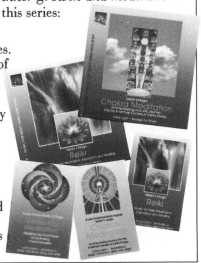

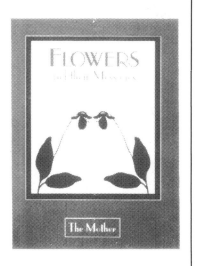
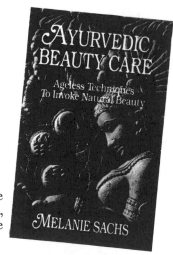